D1927794

INFECTION IN THE NEWBORN

WILEY SERIES ON PERINATAL PRACTICE

Series editors:

Geoffrey Chamberlain
Professor of Obstetrics and Gynaecology,
St George's Hospital Medical School, London, UK

and

Forrester Cockburn
Samson Gemmell Professor of Child Health,
Royal Hospital for Sick Children, Glasgow, UK

Ultrasound in Perinatal Care (out of print)
M.J. Bennett
Professor and Head of School of Obstetrics and Gynaecology,
University of New South Wales, Sydney, Australia

Risks of Labour (out of print)
J.W. Crawford
Department of Obstetrics and Gynaecology,
University of Dundee Medical School, Ninewells Hospital, Dundee, UK

Problems in Obstetric Anaesthesia
Barbara Morgan
Senior Lecturer in Anaesthetics,
Institute of Obstetrics and Gynaecology,
University of London, UK

Parent–Infant Relationships
D. Harvey
Consultant Paediatrician,
Queen Charlotte's Maternity Hospital, London, UK

Fetal and Neonatal Growth
F. Cockburn
Department of Child Health,
Royal Hospital for Sick Children, Glasgow, UK

Infection in the Newborn
J. de Louvois and D. Harvey
Queen Charlotte's and Chelsea Hospital,
London, UK

PERINATAL PRACTICE

Series editors
Geoffrey Chamberlain
Forrester Cockburn

Volume 6

INFECTION IN THE NEWBORN

Editors
John de Louvois and David Harvey
Queen Charlotte's and Chelsea Hospital, London

John Wiley & Sons
Chichester · New York · Brisbane · Toronto · Singapore

Copyright © 1990 by John Wiley & Sons Ltd.
Baffins Lane, Chichester
West Sussex PO19 1UD, England

All rights reserved.

No part of this book may be reproduced by any means, or transmitted, or translated into a machine language without the written permission of the publisher.

Other Wiley Editorial Offices

John Wiley & Sons, Inc., 605 Third Avenue,
New York, NY 10158-0012, USA

Jacaranda Wiley Ltd, G.P.O. Box 859, Brisbane,
Queensland 4001, Australia

John Wiley & Sons (Canada) Ltd, 22 Worcester Road,
Rexdale, Ontario M9W 1L1, Canada

John Wiley & Sons (SEA) Pte Ltd, 37 Jalan Pemimpin 05-04,
Block B, Union Industrial Building, Singapore 2057

Library of Congress Cataloging-in-Publication Data:

Infection in the newborn / edited by John de Louvois and David Harvey.
p. cm.—(Perinatal practice; v. 6)
Includes bibliographical references.
ISBN 0 471 92679 5
1. Communicable diseases in newborn infants. I. De Louvois, John. II. Harvey, David (David Robert) III. Series.
[DNLM: 1. Infant, Newborn, Diseases. 2. Infection—in infancy & childhood. W1 PE788F v.6 / WS 420 I426]
RJ275.I52 1990
618.92′01—dc20
DNLM/DLC
for Library of Congress 89-70738
CIP

British Library Cataloguing in Publication Data

Infection in the newborn.
1. Newborn babies. Diseases
I. De Louvois, John II. Harvey, David
618.9201

ISBN 0 471 92679 5

Phototypeset by Dobbie Typesetting Limited, Tavistock, Devon
Printed by Courier International Limited, Tiptree, Essex

Contents

Contributors

A. J. Barson — *Department of Pathology, St Mary's Hospital, Manchester, UK*

L. Chieco-Bianchi — *Institute of Oncology, University of Padova, Italy*

R. d'Elia — *Department of Paediatrics, University of Padova, Italy*

A. Fleer — *Department of Microbiology, Wilhelmina Children's Hospital, Utrecht, The Netherlands*

L. J. Gerards — *Department of Neonatology, Wilhelmina Children's Hospital, Utrecht, The Netherlands*

C. Giaquinto — *Department of Paediatrics, University of Padova, Italy*

M. A. Hall — *Princess Anne Hospital and Southampton General Hospital, Southampton, UK*

K. N. Haque — *Division of Neonatology, Department of Paediatrics, College of Medicine, Riyadh, Saudi Arabia*

D. R. Harvey — *Department of Paediatrics, Queen Charlotte's and Chelsea Hospital, London, UK*

D. Isaacs — *John Radcliffe Hospital, Oxford, UK*

M. Levin — *The Hospital for Sick Children, Great Ormond Street and the Institute of Child Health, London, UK*

A. B. MacLean — *Department of Obstetrics, Queen Mother's Hospital, Glasgow, Scotland*

J. de Louvois — *Department of Microbiology, Queen Charlotte's and Chelsea Hospital, London, UK*

C. R. Madeley *Department of Clinical Virology, Royal Victoria Infirmary, Newcastle upon Tyne, UK*

A. G. S. Philip *Division of Neonatology, Maine Medical Center, Portland and University of Vermont College of Medicine, USA*

A. de Rossi *Institute of Oncology, University of Padova, Italy*

J. A. D. Spencer *Institute of Obstetrics and Gynaecology, Royal Postgraduate Medical School, University of London and Queen Charlotte's and Chelsea Hospital, London, UK*

F. Zacchello *Department of Paediatrics, University of Padova, Italy*

Series Preface

Obstetrics and neonatal paediatrics have moved closer together in recent years, as they constitute a continuum of care for the fetus and newborn child. Barriers between the two subjects should not exist, because many of the problems of the newborn originate during fetal development, and therefore an understanding of the other half of the problem will help those involved in each discipline. This series is offered as a contribution towards bridging the narrowing gap between obstetrics and neonatal medicine. Each volume contains a series of reviews of topical issues written by specialists in both obstetrics and neonatology, providing the reader with a comprehensive and balanced presentation of current perinatal practice.

Geoffrey Chamberlain
Forrester Cockburn

Preface

Infection continues to be a serious problem for the newborn. As the babies receiving intensive care have become smaller and smaller, the risk of systemic infection has increased. Neonatologists have become used to strange organisms causing overwhelming infection. The techniques of intensive care have become more invasive; central venous catheters or endotracheal tubes are obvious entry routes for germs. Whereas *Candida albicans*, although common, used only to be a cause of oral thrush, it is now recognized as causing septicaemia and subcutaneous abscesses in preterm babies who have received antibiotics and have indwelling catheters.

Not only have new techniques added to the hazards of the newborn, but the bacteria themselves appear to have changed in their ability to invade. The predominant organisms have varied over the last two centuries. The group A streptococcus caused many deaths when the infection was studied by Semmelweiss in Vienna in the 19th century and by Colebrook at Queen Charlotte's Maternity Hospital in the 1930s; it is now uncommon. *Staphylococcus aureus* was common in the 1950s and 1960s but now appears to have been controlled by local antiseptics and antibiotic therapy. In the 1970s infection by *Escherichia coli* gave way to the group B streptococcus (GBS), which has now become greatly feared. The latest organism to appear as a pathogen is *Staphylococcus epidermidis* which is now very commonly found at blood culture. Some organisms, such as *Listeria monocytogenes* and *Toxoplasma gondii* which are much commoner in some countries than others, are currently causing increased concern and may possibly be problems for tomorrow.

Many doctors have been horrified by the rapid death of babies infected with GBS. The only sensible response has been to use antibiotic therapy at once whenever serious infection is suspected. This has the disadvantage that many babies are treated with antibiotics when they are not infected. It is now usual to stop treatment after 48 hours if the baby is well and the cultures are negative, but we are still searching for a way of making an early and definite diagnosis of infection. Fortunately, the recent development of effective and apparently non-toxic antibiotics has allowed us to use treatment widely, but we hope to treat fewer babies in the future.

All of these problems, and others, prompted us to edit this collection of essays on important issues in neonatal infection. They arise from a workshop which was held by the RPMS Institute of Obstetrics and Gynaecology at Brocket Hall. We are grateful for the generous financial support for this workshop provided by the RPMS Institute of Obstetrics and Gynaecology, Glaxo Group Research Ltd, Imperial Chemical Industries Ltd and Cow and Gate Ltd.

John de Louvois
David Harvey

1 The Inflammatory Response to Infections

M. Levin
*The Hospital for Sick Children,
Great Ormond Street and
the Institute of Child Health, London, UK*

Introduction

As a result of widespread awareness of the rapidity with which sepsis may overwhelm the newborn, infection in this age group is usually suspected at the first sign of any illness, and antibiotics are administered. Despite prompt initiation of treatment, and the availability of an ever-increasing armamentarium of potent antibiotics to which the infecting organisms are sensitive, the mortality from neonatal infection remains high (1). It seems unlikely that the prognosis in neonatal infections can be much improved by earlier treatment, or by more potent antibiotics, as the causative organisms are usually sensitive to currently available antimicrobials and are usually rapidly killed by clinically achievable antibiotic concentrations.

This chapter will present the thesis that the infecting agent initiates a pathophysiological process, mediated by the host immune system, which persists after the infecting agent has been killed by antibiotics, and which is responsible for most of the clinical manifestations and organ dysfunction seen in sepsis. Improved prognosis in neonatal infection may come not from more rapid killing of bacteria by antibiotics, but from an understanding of this pathophysiological process and the development of treatments to correct the disordered physiological state.

Triggering of inflammation by infection

Bacteria induce disease by three main mechanisms (2, 3):

(1) by production of extracellular toxins or enzymes which damage host cells and tissue;
(2) by release of cell-wall or intracellular constituents such as endotoxin;
(3) by triggering host inflammatory responses which mediate the tissue damage.

This last mechanism also contributes to damage caused by extracellular toxins and endotoxin (1 and 2).

The clinical picture of neonatal sepsis is familiar to all paediatricians (1). The neonate's skin is pale and mottled, and capillary refill slow. Hypotension may be present and the pulse is rapid and thready. Peripheral perfusion is poor, with a wide gap between central and peripheral temperature. The respirations are rapid or irregular, urine output is low or absent, and the neonate is poorly responsive. Laboratory investigations

Infection in the Newborn. Edited by J. de Louvois and D. Harvey
©1990 John Wiley & Sons Ltd

reveal hypoxia, acidosis, impaired renal function, and hepatic dysfunction. Anaemia, thrombocytopenia and evidence of disseminated intravascular coagulation (DIC) frequently supervene. Later, oedema, jaundice, worsening acidosis, and respiratory and cardiac failure may occur. These familiar clinical features, and the complex multisystem derangement they indicate, are largely the result of three basic processes affecting the vasculature (4, 5):

(1) *Increased vascular permeability.* An alteration in the permeability properties of the vascular endothelium and the capillary wall allows albumin and other colloids to leak from the intravascular space to the interstitial space. This results in hypovolaemia, and diminished venous return to the heart, thereby decreasing cardiac output. Accumulation of extravascular plasma proteins and fluid in the tissues leads to oedema in the pulmonary and other interstitial areas (5, 6).

(2) *Vasoconstriction, or vasodilatation, or both.* Vasoconstriction of arteries and arterioles increases vascular resistance in the systemic and pulmonary circulations, thereby decreasing cardiac output and diminishing perfusion of the kidneys, gastrointestinal tract and other organs. Dilatation of postcapillary venules and some precapillary arterioles results in pooling of blood in the periphery, shunting of blood past some vascular beds, and thus to further reduction in both tissue perfusion and venous return to the heart (4, 5).

(3) *Microvascular obstruction.* Microthrombi composed of platelets, leucocytes and fibrin form within the capillaries of the pulmonary, renal and other vascular beds. A further reduction in organ perfusion occurs, together with the clinical picture of DIC (2, 5–8).

These three basic processes, increased vascular permeability, vasoconstriction/vasodilatation and microvascular obstruction,

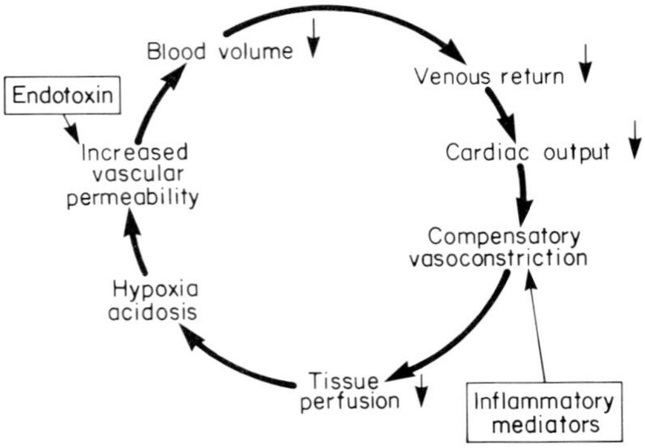

Fig. 1.1. Cyclic mechanisms in septic shock.

produce a pathophysiological cycle which, if maintained, results in septic shock and multiorgan failure (Fig. 1.1). A comprehensive account of the mechanisms by which infectious agents or their toxins initiate these vascular abnormalities is beyond the scope of this chapter. Instead, only some of the inflammatory processes which have recently been recognized, or which offer areas for therapeutic intervention, will be discussed.

The importance of the vascular endothelium

Alterations in the endothelial lining of the vasculature are of key importance in the pathophysiology of sepsis. The vascular endothelial cell is remarkably specialized to maintain vascular homeostasis (9–11): small molecules and water are permitted to pass freely into the tissues, while albumin and larger plasma proteins are confined to the intravascular space; despite passage of blood cells at high speed through narrow capillaries, damage to blood cells is prevented by the non-reactive endothelial surface; platelets and proteins of the coagulation pathway are protected from activation by the non-thrombogenic and platelet inhibitory properties of the endothelium; neutrophils and other inflammatory cells do not normally adhere to the endothelium but readily adhere to and migrate through the endothelium in response to local inflammation. These characteristics of the endothelium are partly due to the intrinsic physicochemical properties of the luminal surface of the endothelium, and in particular to the high concentration of anionic glycosaminoglycans, heparan sulphate and chondroitin sulphate (10, 11). These glycosaminoglycans confer a fixed negative charge on the endothelial surface, and this is important in preventing albumin and other anionic plasma proteins from crossing the endothelial wall and in reducing cellular interaction. Furthermore, the glycosaminoglycans have anticoagulant activities, and also localize several biologically important molecules such as antithrombin III, lipoprotein lipase and platelet factor 4 on the endothelial surface (9, 10). The endothelial cell also maintains vascular homeostasis by actively synthesizing and secreting several important regulatory factors, such as prostacyclin (12), factor VIII, von Willebrand factor and plasminogen activator (9).

The altered vascular permeability, vasoconstriction and intravascular thrombosis seen in sepsis result from a profound alteration in the finely regulated function of the endothelium. The mechanisms by which the endothelium is altered in sepsis and inflammation are currently being intensively investigated and some of this work will be described.

Mediation of the inflammatory response to infection

The role of the macrophages and cytokines

The presence of bacteria, or products released from bacteria into the blood or tissues, triggers an inflammatory response which involves non-cellular effector systems such as complement, kinins and the coagulation pathway, as well as cellular components of the inflammatory system – macrophages, neutrophils, platelets, eosinophils, basophils and lymphocytes (13) (Fig. 1.2).

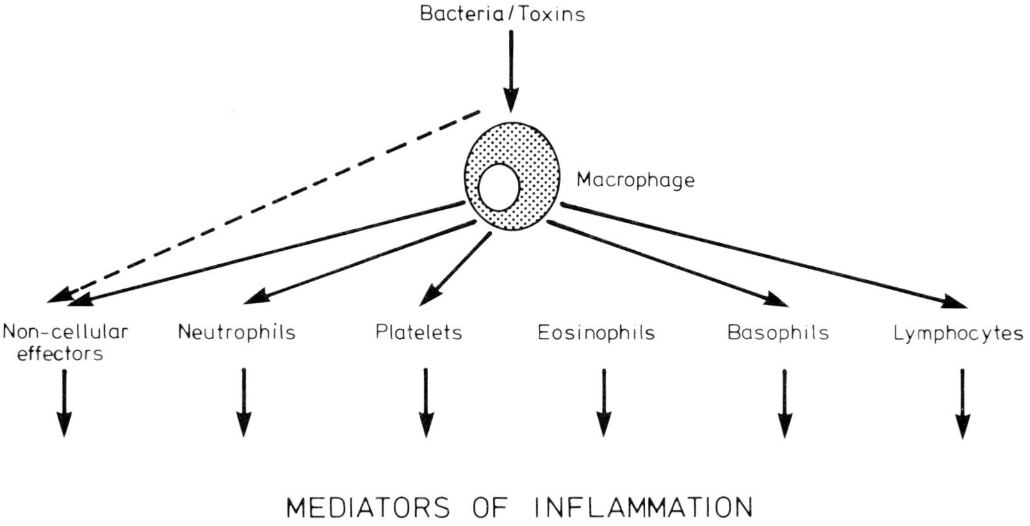

Fig. 1.2. Multiple components of the inflammatory response. Bacteria or their products activate both cellular and non-cellular inflammatory pathways such as complement, kinins and the clotting cascade. The macrophage amplifies the response by releasing cytokines, which in turn activate other cells.

The molecular events by which this response is initiated are not well understood. However, the macrophage probably plays a key role in recognition of the invading microbial organisms and in recruitment of other components of the inflammatory response. The macrophage releases soluble mediators such as interleukin I, tumour necrosis factor (TNF), interferons and platelet activating factor, which activate other inflammatory cells (14). These soluble mediators or cytokines are now thought to be responsible for many of the cellular events occurring in sepsis. In particular, there is growing evidence that TNF may be one of the most important mediators of septic shock.

Tumour necrosis factor has been purified, sequenced and synthesized by recombinant DNA technology. A number of excellent reviews of its biochemistry and physiology have been published (15, 16). Tumour necrosis factor is predominantly released by macrophages, although other cells produce smaller amounts. It is a polypeptide of molecular weight 17 000, which is released in microgram amounts following a variety of stimuli, of which endotoxin is one of the most potent (17). Infusion of TNF into animals induces a state of shock which closely resembles that induced by endotoxin, with hypotension, metabolic acidosis, haemorrhagic infarction of organs and pneumonitis. It is not yet clear whether these effects are directly due to TNF, or are due to activation by TNF of other inflammatory mediators including platelet activating factor and arachidonic-acid metabolites, as some of the effects of TNF can be prevented by inhibiting arachidonic-acid metabolism. Tumour necrosis factor acts on the vascular endothelium to increase neutrophil adherence, procoagulant factor synthesis and suppression of thrombomodulin, thereby favouring thrombus formation on the endothelial surface. This may be relevant to the pathogenesis of DIC. Strong evidence that TNF is important in the pathogenesis of septic shock has come from studies in several different animal species, in which antibodies to TNF were able to prevent mortality and shock in experimental septic or endotoxic shock (16–19).

In addition to cytokines, the macrophage also releases proteins and arachidonic-acid metabolites, which, together with those released from other leucocytes, contribute to vascular and tissue damage (13, 14).

Neutrophils

The role of polymorphonuclear neutrophils in phagocytosing and killing ingested bacteria is well known. Less well known is their function as secretory cells, releasing into the surrounding tissue a variety of potent inflammatory mediators (13, 20). The resting neutrophil has within its cytoplasm numerous granules, containing a variety of biologically active constituents. These include proteolytic enzymes such as elastase, collagenase, myeloperoxidase, cathepsin G and acid hydrolases; several highly cationic proteins; lactoferrin; and vitamin B^{12} binding proteins. These granular constituents are extruded from the neutrophil during activation by a variety of stimuli including phagocytosis; antigen–antibody complexes; activated complement components; and soluble stimulants such as platelet activating factor, leukotrienes and specific peptides (18, 20). In addition to releasing granular constituents, neutrophils activated during infection also release newly synthesized substances such as reactive oxygen intermediates (21), leukotrienes and prostaglandins (13, 20, 21).

Upon activation by phagocytic or soluble stimuli, both neutrophils and macrophages undergo a *respiratory burst*, characterized by an increase in oxygen consumption, activation of the hexose-monophosphate shunt, and generation of reactive oxygen-derived free radicals, superoxide and hydrogen peroxide (H_2O_2). Several other reactive oxygen-derived metabolites are also produced, including hydroxyl radicals and hypochlorous acid. Although most of the oxygen free radicals produced during the respiratory burst are localized within the phagolysosomes, significant amounts also appear extracellularly, and are toxic to endothelial cells, erythrocytes and platelets, as well as damaging to non-cellular proteins (21).

The role of neutrophils in endothelial damage

There is now good evidence that neutrophils can damage endothelial cells during inflammation (22). One of the earliest events in inflammation is adherence of neutrophils to the vascular endothelium (23). The alteration of the endothelial surface which permits adherence of leucocytes can be induced by interleukin 1, complement components or leukotriene B_4 (23, 24), and may serve to bring inflammatory mediators released from neutrophils into close proximity with the endothelium. Several studies have documented that neutrophils stimulated by C5a or specific peptides can lyse endothelial cells (22). The endothelial cell damage is enhanced in the presence of endotoxin, and is probably mediated by both oxygen free radicals and proteolytic enzymes released from the neutrophil (22). Neutrophil-mediated damage to endothelial cells is probably important in endotoxic shock, and in the *shock lung* associated with endotoxaemia (25).

In animal models of endotoxic shock, organ damage can be prevented by neutrophil depletion (26). *In vitro*, neutrophil-mediated endothelial damage can be prevented by specific protease inhibitors and inhibitors of oxygen free radicals, suggesting an important role for proteases and free radicals in endothelial injury (22). The role of neutrophil cationic proteins in altering endothelial permeability is discussed later.

Neutrophil elastase as a mediator of inflammation

There has been increasing interest in the role of proteolytic enzymes released from neutrophils and other inflammatory cells, in mediating endothelial and tissue damage, and initiating intravascular thrombosis in sepsis (27). The danger which proteolytic enzymes present to the body is perhaps indicated by the existence of at least nine plasma proteins, which function to neutralize proteolytic enzymes (28). These plasma protease inhibitors include alpha-1-antitrypsin, antithrombin III, C_1 esterase inhibitor, alpha-2-macroglobulin, antichymotrypsin, alpha-2-plasmin inhibitor, heparin co-factor II and protein C inhibitor. The inhibitors form an inactive complex with their target proteolytic enzyme, which is then cleared from the circulation by the reticuloendothelial system (29). Some of the protease inhibitors, such as alpha-1-antitrypsin and alpha-2-macroglobulin, are able to inactivate several different proteases, whereas others, such as antithrombin III, are more specific in their actions. If proteolytic enzymes are infused into animals experimentally, they are initially neutralized by the protease inhibitors, the concentrations of which decrease. As soon as the protease inhibitors are overwhelmed, and free proteolytic enzymes appear in the circulation, shock, DIC and complement activation occur (30).

In sepsis, release of neutrophil elastase and other proteolytic enzymes in excess of the neutralizing capacity of the plasma protease inhibitors may have similar consequences to that seen in experimental animals. Alpha-1-antitrypsin, the major plasma inhibitor of neutrophil elastase, is an acute-phase reactant, the concentration of which increases in infection, suggesting an important role in regulating the inflammatory response (27). Although alpha-1-antitrypsin is normally present in adequate concentrations to neutralize neutrophil elastase, and localize any elastase to the immediate site of infection, in overwhelming sepsis or endotoxaemia, massive release of neutrophil elastase may overwhelm the protease inhibitors. Furthermore, alpha-1-antitrypsin is inactivated by oxygen free radicals (27, 31). Thus neutrophil-derived reactive oxygen metabolites released during inflammation may inactivate alpha-1-antitrypsin, thereby permitting active proteases to appear in the circulation (Fig. 1.3).

Recent evidence indicates that plasma protease inhibitors such as antithrombin III have a common structure which is susceptible to proteolytic digestion by neutrophil elastase (31). Neutrophil elastase destroys an exposed polypeptide sequence on the inhibitor, which converts it to an inactive form. Thus in inflammation, if elastase is released in sufficient amounts to overwhelm the alpha-1-antitrypsin, elastase may inactivate the inhibitors of coagulation, allowing uncontrolled coagulation and intravascular thrombosis to occur (Fig. 1.4) (27, 31).

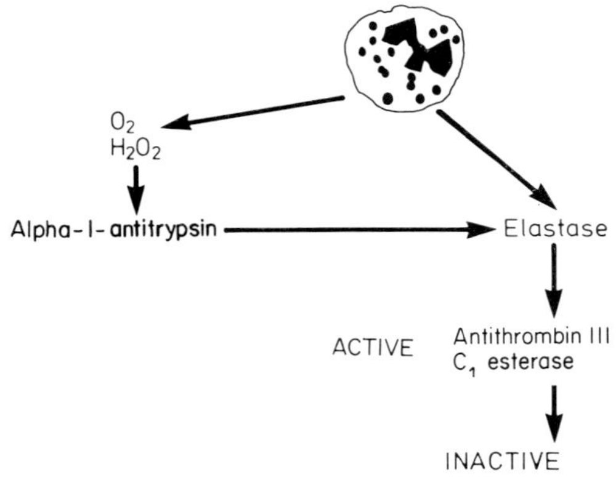

Fig. 1.3. Inactivation of alpha-1-antitrypsin by neutrophil-derived reactive oxygen metabolites. The neutrophil releases both elastase and reactive oxygen metabolites. Alpha-1-antitrypsin, which is normally available to neutralize the elastase, is inactivated by the oxygen free radicals. Free elastase therefore gains access to the circulation and attacks the other protease inhibitors, converting them to inactive forms ($C_1 = C_1$ component of complement).

While this sequence of events has yet to be confirmd in human disease, it is a potentially important mechanism linking neutrophil activation with DIC. Furthermore, it is a pathophysiological sequence which may be interrupted therapeutically. Infusion of fresh frozen plasma, containing protease inhibitors, or purified protease inhibitors such as alpha-1-antitrypsin and antithrombin III, may be beneficial in septic shock and DIC.

Platelets

In addition to their role in thrombosis, platelets are also important in inflammation. Platelets are highly reactive cells which can be activated by a wide range of stimuli including antigen–antibody complexes, platelet activating factor released from macrophages

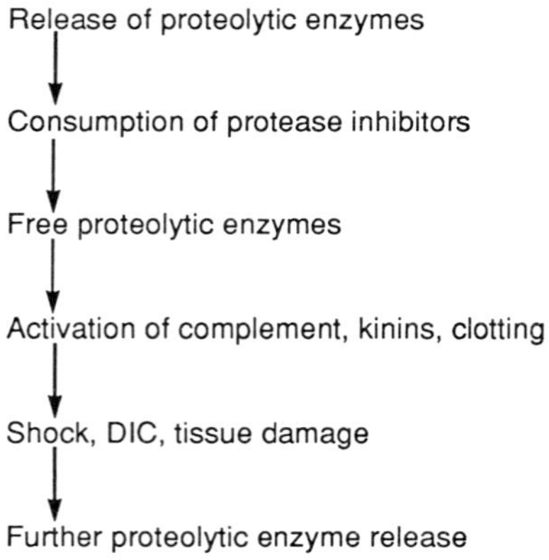

Fig. 1.4. Potential role of proteolytic enzymes in septic shock. Bacteria and toxins cause release of proteolytic enzymes from inflammatory cells. The plasma protease inhibitors are overwhelmed or inactivated. Free proteolytic enzymes appear in the circulation, where they activate complement, kinins and the clotting cascade. In the absence of inhibitors of these pathways, disseminated intravascular coagulation (DIC), capillary leakage and tissue damage ensue.

and leucocytes, thromboxane A_2, thrombin, serotonin, ADP and contact with subendothelial tissues (32, 33). Following activation, the platelets aggregate, adhere to damaged endothelium, and degranulate, releasing into the surrounding plasma a variety of inflammatory mediators, both newly synthesized and stored within the cytoplasmic granules (32–34). Many of the substances released from platelets have important inflammatory properties, and may amplify the inflammatory process by activating other cells and the coagulation pathway. Furthermore, small numbers of aggregated platelets may readily occlude the microvasculature, impairing organ perfusion.

Serotonin, which is actively taken up by platelets and stored within the granules, is released during activation. Serotonin increases vascular permeability, constricts some vascular beds and dilates others, and aggregates other cells (35). Other vasoactive substances released from platelets – adrenaline, thromboxane A_2 and ADP – have vasoconstrictive properties, and also induce aggregation of other platelets (32–34). Platelets also release a number of proteins from their granules during activation: platelet factor 4 has heparin-neutralizing activity and binds to endothelial surfaces; beta-thromboglobulin has antiheparin activity and also depresses prostacyclin production; platelet-derived growth factor stimulates proliferation of subendothelial tissue; and a variety of proteolytic enzymes degrade connective tissue (32–34, 36). There is evidence from both animal studies and human disease that platelet-derived mediators of inflammation contribute to vascular damage in several inflammatory disorders (35–37). Furthermore, inhibition of platelet activation, or antagonism of mediators released from platelets, has a beneficial effect in inflammatory disorders (36, 38). Platelet activation occurs commonly in neonatal sepsis, and inflammatory mediators released from platelets may contribute to the pathophysiological derangement.

Arachidonic-acid metabolism and control of platelet activation

Elucidation of the role played by arachidonic-acid metabolites in vascular homeostasis and inflammation has been one of the major biological advances in the past 20 years (39, 40). Arachidonic acid, the 20-carbon fatty-acid precursor of the prostaglandins, is released from phospholipids in cell walls by the enzyme phospholipase A_2. Arachidonic acid can then undergo metabolism by at least three different pathways, leading to a variety of active metabolites (Fig. 1.5):

(1) via the enzyme cyclo-oxygenase to the prostaglandins, thromboxane and prostacyclin;
(2) via the enzyme lipoxygenase to HPETE and then to the leukotrienes;
(3) via lipoxygenase to the hydroxy-eicosatetraenoic acids (HETEs).

Cyclo-oxygenase converts arachidonic acid initially to unstable intermediary prostaglandins (PGG_2, PGH_2) and then to the prostaglandins (PGE_2, PGF_2), thromboxane A_2 or prostacyclin (PGI_2). The relative amounts of each of these active metabolites produced depends on the tissue or cell involved. Prostacyclin is the major metabolite produced by the vascular endothelial cell. It is the most powerful inhibitor of platelet aggregation, and a potent vasodilator. These platelet inhibiting and vasodilating properties suggest an important role for prostacyclin in preventing intravascular thrombosis and maintaining vascular patency (39, 40). Whereas the endothelial cell preferentially produces prostacyclin, platelets metabolize arachidonic acid to thromboxane A_2, which is a potent vasoconstrictor and platelet-

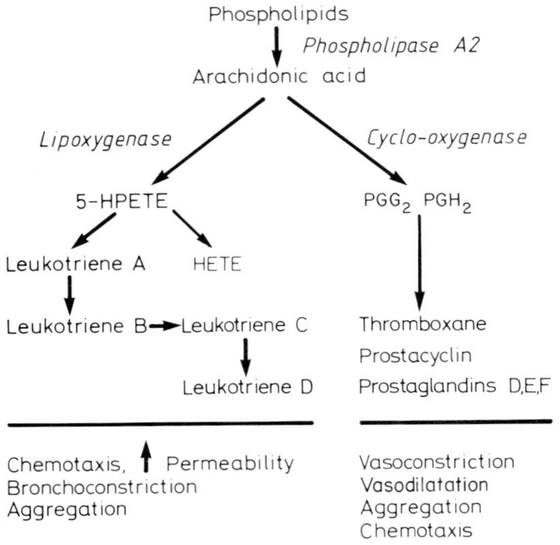

Fig. 1.5. Major metabolic pathways of arachidonic acid metabolism. PGG_2, PGH_2, unstable intermediary prostaglandins; 5-HPETE, hydroperoxy-eicosatetraenoic acid; HETE, hydroxy-eicosatetraenoic acid.

aggregating agent. Smaller amounts of thromboxane are also produced by macrophages and other leucocytes.

The existence of these two metabolites, prostacyclin and thromboxane, with apparently opposing actions, produced by the vessel wall and platelets respectively, has suggested that normal vascular homeostasis depends on a balance between the vasodilating, platelet-inhibiting action of prostacyclin and the vasoconstricting and aggregating effect of thromboxane (39, 40).

Overproduction of thromboxane, which occurs during widespread platelet activation in sepsis, or deficiency of prostacylin production, which occurs after endothelial damage, would result in intravascular thrombosis, vasospasm and release of other inflammatory mediators from platelets. High levels of thromboxane A_2 have been documented in experimental sepsis, and the beneficial effect of prostacyclin infusion or cyclo-oxygenase inhibitors in both experimental sepsis and some human inflammatory disorders suggests that this is an important inflammatory pathway (41, 42).

The prostaglandins (PGE_2, PGF_2, PGD_2) are produced by many cells of the body, including mast cells, neutrophils and macrophages. They have a variety of actions including vasodilation or vasoconstriction, chemotaxis and bronchoconstriction. They are probably important in local regulation of vascular tone and in control of cellular function. The leukotrienes and HETEs are produced by macrophages, neutrophils and monocytes (43). They have powerful inflammatory properties and are important vasoconstrictors, bronchoconstrictors and chemotactic agents (41, 43).

Leukotriene B_4 is a potent chemotactic agent, and also induces degranulation of neutrophils. Leukotrienes C_4, D_4 and E_4 have bronchoconstrictor activity, constrict other smooth muscles and increase vascular permeability, and are probably responsible for the activity previously known as slow-reacting substances of anaphylaxis. Release of leukotrienes and HETEs from leucocytes during inflammation may thus be important in the pathogenesis of the vasoconstriction, increased permeability and intravascular aggregation of cells (42, 43).

The availability of pharmacological agents which interfere with prostaglandin or leukotriene production or action, offers several areas for therapeutic intervention (39, 42, 43). Steroids inhibit arachidonic-acid metabolism by reducing the activity of phospholipase A_2. Aspirin and other non-steroidal anti-inflammatory drugs inhibit cyclo-oxygenase, thus blocking production of prostaglandins. Cells vary in their sensitivity to cyclo-oxygenase inhibitors, with lower doses inhibiting platelet cyclo-oxygenase, and higher doses endothelial cyclo-oxygenase (39). It is therefore possible to inhibit selectively thromboxane synthesis while leaving prostacyclin production intact. Specific inhibitors of thromboxane synthesis are already in clinical use, but clinically useful lipoxygenase inhibitors are not currently available, although they may be in the future (42, 44). Prostacyclin is already being used as a vasodilator and platelet-inhibiting agent to treat a variety of disorders including septic shock (45, 46). Although there have so far been few attempts to correct the pathophysiological derangements in sepsis by administration of drugs which alter arachidonic-acid metabolism, this is a promising area for research, and there are preliminary studies suggesting beneficial effects of prostaglandin inhibitors or prostacyclin in both experimental and human inflammatory disorders (39, 44–46).

Vascular permeability and the role of cationic proteins

Increased vascular permeability to albumin and other plasma proteins is an important feature of sepsis, and results in hypovolaemia and interstitial oedema. Several different mechanisms may cause the increase in vascular permeability, including endothelial cell destruction, opening of interendothelial gaps and damage to the basement membrane, mediated by histamine, serotonin, leukotrienes, proteolytic enzymes or the kinin pathway (6, 7). However, an additional mechanism which has received attention recently is an alteration in the negative charge on the endothelial cell and basement membrane (10, 11, 47).

The luminal surface of endothelial cells and the basement membrane are highly negatively charged due to the presence of the anionic glycosaminoglycans, heparan sulphate, chondroitin sulphate and dermatan sulphate, in the glycoproteins of the cell membrane (10, 11). It is now well established that albumin and other anionic plasma proteins are retained within the vascular space not only by their size, which limits their passage across the capillary wall, but also by their charge (47). An electrostatic repulsion between albumin and other plasma proteins which are negatively charged at physiological pH, and the negative charge on the endothelial surface, prevents passage of the proteins across the capillary wall. Reduction of the negative charge on the endothelial cell, either by enzymatic degradation of the glycosaminoglycans, or following their neutralization by polycations, results in increased vascular permeability (11, 47, 48). Many cells of the inflammatory system including macrophages (49), platelets (50), neutrophils (51) and eosinophils (51) contain highly cationic proteins, which are released during activation of the cells. These cationic proteins are known to increase vascular permeability (50, 51), as well as having opsonic, heparin-neutralizing and bactericidal activities (49, 50).

Cationic proteins released from inflammatory cells during sepsis may bind to and neutralize the negative charge on the endothelial cells and basement membranes, thereby reducing the capillary-wall negative charge and increasing the permeability to albumin. Neutralization of endothelial cell negative charge by cationic proteins has been demonstrated in experimentally induced inflammation, and also in human disease such as systemic lupus erythematosis (52, 53). If similar mechanisms occur in sepsis, administration of highly anionic substances such as heparan sulphate may help to neutralize the cationic proteins and restore the capillary-wall negative charge.

Clinical significance of the inflammatory response in sepsis

Some of the inflammatory mediators responsible for the physiological derangement seen in septic shock have been discussed in this chapter. It seems likely that pharmacological agents which prevent the synthesis or release of these inflammatory mediators, or which reverse their effects, may be useful in treating sepsis. Furthermore, antibodies (either monoclonal or polyclonal) directed against bacterial products such as endotoxin, or against inflammatory mediators, may prevent or reverse the pathophysiological process induced by bacteria. Antibodies against TNF have already been shown to be beneficial in animal models of septic shock, and trials in patients are already under way (17, 19).

Further study of the mechanisms involved in septic shock will no doubt provide other sites for therapeutic intervention, either by pharmacological or by immunological agents.

In view of the continued mortality and morbidity from neonatal sepsis, despite early antibiotic administration and intensive care, trials of inflammation-modulating therapy are clearly warranted. Table 1.1 shows some of the therapeutic agents available which modulate the inflammatory response or reverse the vasoconstriction, bronchoconstriction and increased vascular permeability seen in sepsis. As the pathophysiology of sepsis becomes better understood, these and other inflammation-modulating drugs are likely to become important adjuncts to the treatment of overwhelming infection.

Table 1.1. *Therapeutic possibilities*

Inhibitors of mediators	Cyclo-oxygenase inhibitors Lipoxygenase inhibitors Corticosteroids
Receptor-blocking agents	Kentanserin (serotonin blocking agent) Phentolamine PAF inhibitors
Physiological antagonists	Vasodilators Prostacyclin Beta-agonists
Protease inhibitors	Alpha-1-antitrypsin Antithrombin III
Antioxidants	Superoxide dysmutase O_2 scavengers
Monoclonal antibodies	Anti-endotoxin Anti-TNF

PAF, platelet activating factor; TNF, tumour necrosis factor.

References

1. McCracken GH, Friej B. Infectious diseases of the fetus and newborn. In: Cherry JD, Feigin RD (eds) Textbook of pediatric infectious diseases. 2nd ed. Philadelphia: WB Saunders, 1987: 940–966.
2. Morrison DC, Ulevitch RJ. The effect of bacterial endotoxins on host mediation systems. Am J Pathol 1978; 93: 527–617.
3. Hewlett EL. Microbial virulence factors. In: Mandell GL, Douglas RG, Bennett JE (eds) Principles and practice of infectious diseases. New York: Wiley, 1985: 2–25.
4. Blain CM, Anderson TO, Pietras RJ. Immediate haemodynamic effects of gram-negative vs gram-positive bacteraemia. Arch Intern Med 1970; 126: 260–5.
5. Levin M. Pathogenesis and treatment of shock. In: Black J (ed.) Paediatric emergencies . 2nd ed. London: Butterworth, 1987: 87–116.
6. Anderson RR, Holliday RL, Driedgen AA. Documentation of pulmonary capillary permeability in adult respiratory distress syndrome accompanying human sepsis. Am Rev Respir Dis 1979; 119: 869–77.
7. Christy JH. Pathophysiology of gram-negative shock. Am Heart J 1971; 81: 694–701.
8. Rodriguez-Erdmann F. Intravascular activation of the clotting system with phospholipids. Blood 1965; 26: 451–5.
9. Wall RT, Harker LA. The endothelium and thrombosis. Ann Rev Med 1980; 31: 361–70.
10. Wight TN. Vessel proteoglycan and thrombogenesis. In: Spaet TH (ed.) Progress in hemostasis and thrombosis, vol. 5. New York: Grune and Stratton, 1980: 1–39.
11. Kanwar YS. Biophysiology of glomerular filtration and proteinuria. Lab Invest 1984; 51: 7–21.
12. Moncada S, Vane JR. Prostacyclin: its biosynthesis, actions and clinical potential. Phil Trans R Soc Lond 1981; B294: 305–29.

13. Dale MM, Foreman JC (eds). Textbook of immunopharmacology. Oxford: Blackwell Scientific, 1987.
14. Nathan CF. Secretory products of macrophages. J Clin Invest 1987; 79: 319–26.
15. Beutler B, Cerami A. Tumour necrosis, cachexia, shock and inflammation: a common mediator. Ann Rev Biochem 1988; 57: 505–18.
16. Beutler B, Cerami A. Cachectin, cachexia and shock. Ann Rev Med 1988; 39: 75–83.
17. Mathison JC, Wolfson E, Ulevitch RJ. Participation of tumor necrosis factor in the mediation of gram-negative bacterial lipopolysaccharide induced injury in rabbits. J Clin Invest 1988; 81: 1925–37.
18. Tracey KF, Fong Y, Hesse DG, Manogue KR, Lee AT, Cerami A. Anti-cachectin/TNF monoclonal antibodies prevent septic shock during lethal bacteraemia. Nature 1987; 330: 662–4.
19. Shimamoto Y, Chen RL, Bollon A, Chang A, Khan A. Monoclonal antibodies against recombinant tumor necrosis factor: prevention of endotoxic shock. Immunol Lett 1988; 17: 311–18.
20. Klebanoff SJ, Clark RA. The neutrophil: functional and clinical disorders. Amsterdam: North Holland, 1978.
21. Fantone FC, Ward R. Role of oxygen-derived free radicals and metabolites in leukocyte-dependent inflammatory reactions. Am J Pathol 1982; 107: 394–418.
22. Smedly LA, Tonnesen MG, Sandhaus RA. Neutrophil mediated injury to endothelial cells. J Clin Invest 1986; 77: 1233–43.
23. Harlan JM. Leukocyte–endothelial interactions. Blood 1985; 65: 513–25.
24. Bevilacqua M, Pober J, Wheeler M, Cotran RS, Gimbrone MA. Interleukin I acts on cultured human vascular endothelium to increase adhesion of polymorphonuclear leukocytes, monocytes and related leukocyte cell lines. J Clin Invest 1985; 76: 2003–11.
25. Repine JE, Bowman CM, Tate RM. Neutrophils and lung oedema: state of the art. Am Rev Respir Dis 1982; 81: 47–50.
26. Heflin AC, Brigham KL. Prevention by granulocyte depletion of increased vascular permeability of sheep lung following endotoxaemia. J Clin Invest 1981; 68: 1253–60.
27. Carrell RW. α_1 antitrypsin. Molecular pathology: leukocytes and tissue damage. J Clin Invest 1986; 78: 1427–31.
28. Harpel PC. Protease inhibitors – a precarious balance. New Engl J Med 1983; 309: 725–6.
29. Travis J, Salvesen GS. Human plasma proteinase inhibitors. Ann Rev Biochem 1983; 52: 655–709.
30. Kwaan HC, Anderson MC, Gramatica L. A study of pancreatic enzymes as a factor in the pathogenesis of disseminated intravascular coagulation during acute pancreatitis. Surgery 1971; 69: 663–72.
31. Carrell RW, Owen MC. Plakalbumin, α_1 antitrypsin, antithrombin and the mechanisms of inflammatory thrombosis. Nature 1985; 317: 730–2.
32. Nachman RL, Polley M. The platelet as an inflammatory cell. Trans Am Clin Climatol Assoc 1979; 90: 38–43.
33. Gordon JL. Platelets in biology and pathology. In: Douglas JT, Gordon JL (eds) Research monographs in cell and tissue physiology, vol. 5. Amsterdam: Elsevier/North Holland, 1981.
34. George CRP, Clark WF, Cameron JS. The role of platelets in glomerulonephritis. Adv Nephrol 1975; 5: 19–65.
35. Parbtani A, Frampton G, Cameron JS. Platelet and plasma serotonin concentrations in glomerulonephritis II. Clin Nephrol 1980; 14: 112–16.
36. Cameron JS. Platelets in glomerular disease. Ann Rev Med 1984; 35: 175–80.
37. Levin M, Holland PC, Nokes TJC, Novelli V, Dillon MJ, Barratt TM, Marshall WC. Platelet immune complex interaction in the pathogenesis of Kawasaki disease and childhood polyarteritis. Br Med J 1985; 290: 1456–60.
38. Cochrane CG. Mechanisms involved in the deposition of immune complexes in tissue. J Exp Med 1971; 134: 755–8.
39. Wu KK, Rossi EC (eds). Prostaglandins in clinical medicine: cardiovascular and thrombotic disorders. London: Year Book, 1981.
40. Moncada S, Vane JR. Unstable metabolites of arachidonic acid and their role in haemostasis and thrombosis. Br Med Bull 1978; 34: 129–36.
41. Flohe L, Giertz H. Endotoxins: arachidonic acid and superoxide formations. Rev Inf Dis 1987; 9: 553–61.
42. Schrauwen E, Vandeplassche G, Laekeman G, Houvenaghel A. Endotoxic shock in piglets: beneficial effects of prostaglandin synthesis inhibition. Prostagl Leukotr Med 1984; 13: 271–8.
43. Samuelsson B. Leukotrienes: mediators of immediate hypersensitivity reactions and inflammation. Science 1983; 220: 568–75.

44. Goldberg RN, Suguihara C, Streitfeld M, Baracalari A, Baracalari E. Effects of a leukotriene antagonist on the early haemodynamic manifestations of group B streptococcal sepsis in piglets. Ped Res 1987; 20: 1004–8.
45. Bihari D, Simmons M, Gordon A, Tinker J. The effects of vasodilatation with prostacyclin on oxygen delivery and uptake in critically ill patients. N Engl J Med 1987; 327: 1483–7.
46. Bihari DJ, Tinker J. The therapeutic value of vasodilator prostaglandins in multiple organ failure associated with sepsis. Intens Care Med 1988; 15: 3–7.
47. Brenner BM, Hostetter TH, Humes, HD. Molecular basis of proteinuria of glomerular origin. N Engl J Med 1978; 298: 826–33.
48. Vehaskari VM, Chang CT, Stevens JK, Robson AM. The effects of polycations on vascular permeability in the rat: a proposed role for charge sites. J Clin Invest 1984; 73: 1053–61.
49. Patterson-Delafield J, Martinez RJ, Lehrer RI. Microbicidal cationic proteins in rabbit alveolar macrophages: a potential host defense mechanism. Infect Immun 1980; 30: 180–92.
50. Nachman RL, Weskler B, Ferris B. Characterisation of human platelet vascular permeability enhancing activity. J Clin Invest 1972; 51: 549–56.
51. Olsson I, Olofsson T, Venge P, Winquist I. Release of biologically active compounds from neutrophil and eosinophil leukocyte granules. Monogr Allergy 1981; 17: 130–47.
52. Camussi G, Tetta C, Segoloni RC, Vercellone A. Localisation of neutrophil cationic proteins and loss of anionic charges in glomeruli of patients with systemic lupus erythematosus glomerulonephritis. Clin Immun Immunopath 1982; 24: 299–314.
53. Cammussi G, Tetta C, Coda R, Segoloni G, Vercelloni A. Platelet activating factor induced loss of glomerular anionic charges. Kidney Int 1984; 25: 73–81.

2 A Postmortem Study of Infection in the Newborn from 1976 to 1988

A. J. Barson
Department of Pathology, St Mary's Hospital Manchester, UK

Summary

A review is made of the incidence and nature of infection diagnosed from histopathological examination of tissues from 1336 infants dying in a maternity hospital with a regional intensive care unit. These comprised 434 stillbirths, 779 neonatal and 123 postneonatal deaths. Only 1.8% of the stillbirths were infected. Necropsies on the liveborn infants demonstrated pneumonia in 27.9%, septicaemia in 13.4%, necrotizing enterocolitis (NEC) in 5.5%, peritonitis without NEC in 4.7% and meningitis in 3.0%. Systemic candidiasis occurred in 3.7% and cytomegalovirus in 1.2%. *Escherichia coli* was the most commonly isolated pathogen at all sites, but streptococci were seen frequently in the pneumonia and meningitis groups. Coagulase-negative staphylococci were common in septicaemia and NEC. Infection was the main cause of death once survival of the premature infant had been extended long enough for the adverse effects of birth asphyxia and lack of surfactant to decline. Neonatal infections had a strong iatrogenic background among which mechanical ventilation, catheterization, parenteral nutrition and multiple antibiotic exposure were important components.

Introduction

Any doctor's insight into infection in the newborn is determined, like all other aspects of medicine, by his own experience. Obstetricians, neonatologists and pathologists, by virtue of the blinkers which have to be worn in the practice of their respective disciplines, are each confined to particular facets of a common problem.

The bulk of the literature on infection derives largely from those with responsibility for treating it (1–3), and the proliferation of intensive care units for the newborn and their increasing technological sophistication have done nothing to lessen interest in the subject (4–6). Indeed, it has become apparent that the major advances made in getting immature infants to cope with extrauterine existence have not been accompanied by a similar ability to help these infants either to avoid or to survive the hazards of infection.

To the dispassionate eye of the pathologist the modern intensive care unit for the newborn seems almost designed to court the opportunistic ingenuity of micro-organisms. The patients on such a unit are born of mothers who are commonly infected and through birth canals which are impossible to sterilize. The infants are kept warm and moist,

Infection in the Newborn. Edited by J. de Louvois and D. Harvey
©1990 John Wiley & Sons Ltd

wrapped in aluminium foil and enclosed in transparent plastic incubators, so that any organism trapped within may be anticipated to grow vigorously. Bacteria may be provided with direct access to the patient's lungs via the humidified gases of an endotracheal tube or to the aortic blood via an umbilical arterial catheter. Often several incubators are located in one room, so that staff may transfer bacteria from one to another and infected infants who are discharged leave behind a reservoir of organisms for the next uninfected admission. Perhaps overriding all these considerations, and differentiating the circumstances from those seen on the adult intensive care unit, is the fact that the infants are immature, with immunological defences intrinsically incapable of providing adequate protection. The predicament of the very immature is not wholly unlike that of the adult with AIDS. Pathogens do not discriminate between patients who have not acquired immunity and those who have lost it.

The disadvantage of morbid anatomy as a discipline is that the practitioner is less aware of the incidence of infection among those patients who survive. On the other hand the paediatrician who is ignorant of the pathology has a severely distorted view of reality. After necropsy the clinical diagnosis has to be changed or significantly supplemented in a quarter to half of all perinatal deaths (7, 8). Despite this there have been relatively few specifically pathological enquiries which have defined the incidence of infection in perinatal deaths. The broadest-based investigation into the incidence of infection was included as part of the British Birth Surveys of 1958 and 1970 (9, 10), which reviewed necropsies on 2343 stillbirths and neonatal deaths in the UK in March 1958. In terms of size the only comparable study was a retrospective review of 2000 perinatal deaths in Melbourne between 1961 and 1966 (11), although there have been several smaller morbid anatomical investigations since (12–16). The present study is an assessment of the incidence and nature of infection found between 1976 and 1988 in the course of 1336 infant postmortem examinations in a maternity hospital with a regional intensive care unit.

Table 2.1. *Annual incidence of necropsies on stillbirths, neonatal and postneonatal deaths*

Year	Stillbirths		Neonatal deaths		Postneonatal deaths	
	Inborn	Outborn	Inborn	Outborn	Inborn	Outborn
1976	52	0	32	16	1	2
1977	39	0	29	25	4	2
1978	32	0	37	49	5	2
1979	29	2	39	44	4	5
1980	35	1	42	45	8	1
1981	25	2	16	32	5	6
1982	26	5	27	40	3	5
1983	24	6	27	21	8	8
1984	22	3	26	30	1	10
1985	19	5	27	34	5	6
1986	26	10	29	22	10	6
1987	27	17	26	23	8	5
1988	15	12	21	20	2	1
Total	371	63	378	401	64	59
Total inborn plus outborn	434		779		123	

Material and methods

During the 13-year period from 1976 to 1988 there were 56 991 births in St Mary's Hospital. Among these there were 403 stillbirths (a stillbirth rate of 7.1 per 1000), on whom there were 371 necropsies (92%). There were 486 neonatal deaths among infants born in St Mary's Hospital, 378 (78%) of whom were examined *post mortem*. There were 430 first-week deaths during the study, giving a perinatal mortality rate of 14.6 per 1000. Infants born outside the hospital but dying after admission to the regional intensive care unit accounted for 401 neonatal necropsies. Postneonatal necropsies comprised 64 inborn and 59 outborn infants. Postmortem examinations were also made on 63 stillbirths from outside hospitals who were referred to the pathologist for an opinion. The annual incidence of these necropsies is set out in Table 2.1. There has been a decline in the number of stillbirths during the period of the study, although referral of stillbirths has become more common. There is some indication that postneonatal deaths have increased at the expense of the neonatal deaths. The total of 1336 necropsies excludes sudden home deaths and deaths in chronically sick children dying after admission from home.

With regard to the taking of microbiological specimens, the only rigid rule during the period of the study was that a block of lung tissue was always sent to the bacteriology laboratory. Swabs were taken routinely from the interior of lung tissue after searing the surface. The taking of other specimens was left to the discretion of the pathologist. In practice, intracardiac blood cultures were taken from nearly all infants dying in the intensive care unit or where there was a history of maternal pyrexia. Cerebrospinal fluid (CSF) from cisternal puncture was always cultured where there was any clinical or pathological suspicion of meningitis. Placental tissue, if available, was cultured whenever there was reasonable suspicion that the amniotic fluid was infected or that the mother was pyrexial at delivery. Intracardiac blood was always taken immediately after opening the thorax, before dissection of the thoracic organs. All bacteriological samples were cultured both aerobically and anaerobically.

Specimens were rarely sent for virological culture, and then only when there was good clinical indication that the result might be positive. Cytomegalovirus infection was usually diagnosed solely on histopathological grounds.

It is important to emphasize that the diagnosis of infection in this study was based primarily on histopathological evidence. Bacteriological culture was used only in a confirmatory role or to identify specifically the pathogen involved. Positive bacterial cultures, taken *post mortem*, were ignored in the absence of appropriate histopathology, because of the impossibility of distinguishing between postmortem contamination and infection occurring too soon before death for an inflammatory cellular response to become manifest. Due weight was given to a history of positive blood culture during life, even in the absence of a positive blood culture after death, because of the inhibiting effect of antibiotics on laboratory culture. Pathological and bacteriological evidence of inflammation in the placenta was discounted unless there was histological inflammation in fetal organs.

Results

Stillbirths

Eight of 434 (1.8%) stillbirths had histological evidence of infection in fetal tissue (Table 2.2). Four of these infants had acute inflammatory cell consolidation of the lungs, indicative of intrauterine pneumonia (Fig. 2.1). *Streptococcus viridans* was cultured from

Table 2.2. *Stillbirths with histological evidence of infection*

Infection	Gestation (weeks)	Body weight (g)	Acute amnionitis	Prolonged rupture of membranes
Pneumonia	40	2700	Yes	No
Pneumonia	42	3600	No	No
Pneumonia	36	1900	Yes	Yes
Pneumonia	41	3100	Yes	No
Listeriosis	38	2900	Yes	No
Listeriosis	33	1300	No	No
Cytomegalovirus	41	2900	No	Yes
Cytomegalovirus	36	2300	No	No

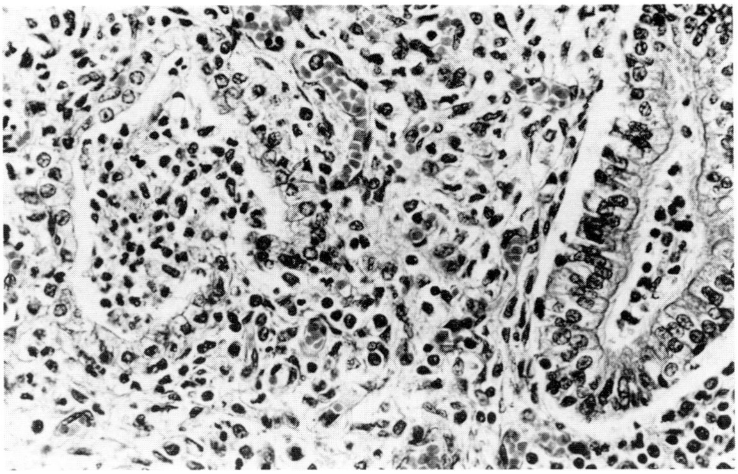

Fig. 2.1. Acute inflammatory cells filling an alveolus on the left and a bronchiole on the right in a stillborn infant. (Stain: haematoxylin and eosin. Magnification: ×350.)

the lung of one, but no organism was grown from the other three although streptococci were identified histologically in one. Three were associated with an acute amnionitis, and in one of these cases the membranes had been ruptured for 2 days.

There were two cases of listeriosis. One of the infants concerned was growth retarded, and characteristic gram-positive bacilli were identified in periadrenal fat. The organism was cultured from intracardiac blood but not from the placenta. The other had an intra-uterine peritonitis and an acute amnionitis in which the organism was seen and cultured.

Cytomegalic inclusions were present in the kidney and lungs of two stillbirths. One of these also had inclusions in the liver. Virological cultures were not undertaken. The birth of one infant had involved prolonged rupture of the membranes.

In addition to these eight cases of definite intrauterine infection there were five suspicious cases. Two of these had multiple small calcific foci, one in the liver and spleen and the other in the kidney. Such lesions may be seen after a viraemic infection has organized, but they are not specific (Fig. 2.2). One patient had had rubella, although the

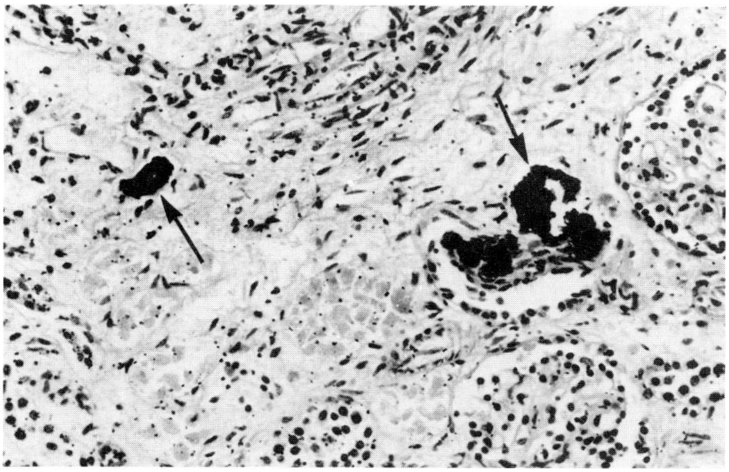

Fig. 2.2. Calcific foci (arrowed) in the kidney of a macerated stillborn infant. (Stain: haematoxylin and eosin. Magnification: ×350.)

virus was never cultured, and the other stillbirth had a cataract in addition to the calcific foci but no history of maternal rubella or positive culture. Another case of maternal rubella resulted in a stillbirth with renal agenesis. One mother was treated for a gonococcal infection at 15 weeks. Her fetus was chronically growth retarded and was stillborn at 30 weeks with absence of one adrenal. The remaining case was also growth retarded with focal renal calcification and a histiocytic infiltration of the intervillus spaces suggestive of a viral infection, although this could not be proved.

Live births

The necropsies on the liveborn infants revealed five major categories of infection which either were in themselves fatal or at least were a major component in the cause of death. These categories are not mutually exclusive. They are listed in Table 2.3. A total of 902 necropsies on liveborn infants revealed 492 serious infections in 383 babies.

Table 2.3. *Incidence of major categories of infection in 902 necropsies on liveborn infants and in 383 infected necropsies among these infants*

Infection	Number of necropsies	Percentage of all necropsies	Percentage of all infected necropsies
Pneumonia	252	27.9	65.8
Septicaemia	121	13.4	31.6
NEC	50	5.5	13.1
Peritonitis*	42	4.7	11.0
Meningitis	27	3.0	7.1
Total	492		

NEC, necrotizing enterocolitis.
*Excludes NEC.

Bronchopneumonia

Table 2.4 divides 252 cases of bronchopneumonia into those dying on the first day, and early, late and postneonatal deaths. The diagnosis was made in all these infants on the basis of acute inflammatory cell consolidation in the alveoli seen in histological sections. It was routine to take at least one block from

Table 2.4. *Relationship of pathology to survival in 252 infants dying with bronchopneumonia*

Survival (days)	0–1	1–7	8–28	29+
Total numbers	62	83	41	66
HMD	47%	60%	29%	9%
BPD	—	12%	49%	38%
Mean gestation (weeks)	31	34	32	32
Mean dead weight (g)	1693	2093	1558	2259
Blood culture +ve	23%	28%	71%	62%
Lung culture +ve	60%	57%	78%	70%

HMD, hyaline membrane disease; BPD, bronchopulmonary dysplasia.

Table 2.5. *Lung cultures from 252 infants dying with pneumonia*

	Number of necropsies			
Organism	0–1	1–7	8–28	29+
No growth	25	36	10	23
Escherichia coli	12	8	3	18
Group B streptococcus	7	2	0	1
Other haemolytic streptococci	2	2	0	3
Non-haemolytic streptococci	3	3	3	8
Streptococcus viridans	3	7	2	4
Streptococcus pneumoniae	1	0	0	1
Anaerobic streptococci	3	0	0	0
Bacteroides sp.	2	2	1	0
Coagulase-negative staphylococci	4	11	3	4
Staphylococcus aureus	2	7	1	3
Staphylococcus epidermidis	0	0	0	1
Pseudomonas sp.	3	6	14	12
Haemophilus sp.	4	2	0	0
Enterobacter sp.	0	4	0	1
Clostridium sp.	0	1	2	1
Proteus sp.	0	2	0	1
Citrobacter sp.	0	1	1	2
Klebsiella sp.	0	0	1	6
Serratia marcescens	0	0	1	1
Mycoplasma sp.	1	0	0	0
Candida sp.	0	0	4	10
Total with pneumonia	62	83	41	66

each lung and commonly more. No attempt was made to grade the severity of the pneumonia or assess its importance to the causation of death relative to other diseases present. The overall tendency is for factors causing death to multiply with postnatal survival and for opinion as to the main cause of death to become correspondingly more subjective. In all these infants the degree of histopathological change in the lungs led the histopathologist to believe that bronchopneumonia was an important factor underlying the infant's death.

It may be seen from Table 2.4 that not all had positive lung cultures despite the morphological diagnosis of pneumonia, although the proportion of positive lung cultures increased with postnatal survival. A significant proportion of these infants dying with bronchopneumonia also had positive intracardiac blood cultures, the proportion increasing from 28% to 71% after the first postnatal week.

The great majority of these infants were born prematurely and received ventilatory support because of respiratory distress syndrome. It was therefore common for pneumonia to be associated with histopathological evidence of hyaline membrane disease or bronchopulmonary dysplasia (Table 2.4). As would be expected, the former pathology declined with survival and the latter increased.

Lung culture was attempted in all 252 infants, and the organisms grown in the four survival groups are shown in Table 2.5. Many cultures grew more than one organism. Although great care was taken in the collection of the cultures, it is impossible to be certain how many of the organisms grown were contaminants. *Escherichia coli* was the bacterium most frequently isolated. Because the diagnosis of pneumonia was made on histological grounds, and because it takes up to 24 h for inflammatory cells to accumulate into significant exudate, it is reasonable to assume that the great majority of those infants dying on the first postnatal day with bronchopneumonia acquired their infecting pathogen *in utero* or whilst passing through the birth canal. Infections with the group B haemolytic streptococcus, anaerobic streptococci and *Bacteroides* sp. were all probably prenatal in origin. Of 18 isolates of these organisms, 12 were from infants dying on the first day and 16 were from infants dying during the first week. On the other hand *Pseudomonas* sp., *Klebsiella* sp. and *Candida* sp. predominated in those infants dying with pneumonia after the first postnatal week. Out of the 62 infants dying with pneumonia on the first day of life, the placenta was available for examination in 14. Histological acute chorioamnionitis was seen in 11 of these cases, again suggesting an intrauterine origin for the infection.

Septicaemia

The diagnosis of septicaemia after death cannot rest on any single criterion. Purely morphological grounds for the diagnosis are evident only in a minority of infants. Multiple disseminated abscesses of similar size, purulent vasculitis and intravascular identification of bacteria are helpful in this respect. Opinion must also take into account postmortem intracardiac blood culture, although of the 121 cases whose cultures are recorded in Table 2.6 four infants had negative postmortem blood cultures. However, the diagnosis of septicaemia was made unequivocally in these infants.

Supportive but not conclusive evidence of a septicaemia may be derived from a postmortem diagnosis of disseminated intravascular coagulopathy. This may take the form of strands of interlacing fibrin seen in the vessels of many organs, but particularly the lung (Fig. 2.3). This was seen in 42 (35%) of the cases. Alternatively, the presence of a well-demarcated subarachnoid fibrinous haematoma may also indicate intravascular coagulopathy (Fig. 2.4). Subarachnoid haematomata were seen in 27 (22%) of the series. Although disseminated intravascular coagulopathy at this age is commonly a product of septicaemia, it cannot be assumed to be diagnostic by itself. Among the 781 necropsies on liveborn infants without septicaemia there were a further 32 (4%) instances of intravascular fibrin and 17 (2%) cases of subarachnoid haematomata (Table 2.7).

Table 2.6. *Blood cultures from 121 infants dying with septicaemia*

Organism	Number of necropsies
E. coli	36
Coagulase-negative staphylococci	23
Candida sp.	19
Pseudomonas sp.	15
Staph. aureus	9
Group B streptococcus	7
Klebsiella sp.	7
Clostridium sp.	6
Enterobacter sp.	5
Non-haemolytic streptococci	5
Citrobacter sp.	4
Enterococcus	4
Strep. viridans	4
Acinetobacter sp.	2
Bacteroides sp.	2
Haemolytic streptococci group D	2
Serratia sp.	2
Proteus sp.	1
Staph. epidermidis	1
Strep. faecium	1
Strep. pneumoniae	1
Total isolates from 121 infants	156

The four most common pathogens grown in blood culture were *E. coli*, coagulase-negative staphylococci, *Candida* sp. and *Pseudomonas* sp. (Table 2.6). These organisms accounted for 93 (60%) of 156 isolates from the 121 infants with septicaemia. Nearly all cases of septicaemia were derived from infants nursed on the intensive care unit. The number of infants dying with septicaemia has increased over the 11 years of the study (Table 2.8). This is probably a reflection of the increasing immaturity of those receiving treatment and their longer survival.

Table 2.7. *Incidence of disseminated intravascular coagulopathy and subarachnoid haematoma in septicaemic and control groups*

	Number (and %) of cases	
	Positive blood culture	Negative blood culture
Total cases	121	781
Disseminated intravascular coagulopathy	42 (34.7)	32 (4.1)
Subarachnoid haematoma	27 (22.3)	17 (2.2)

Table 2.8. *Annual incidence of different forms of sepsis among deaths in liveborn infants*

	Number of cases												
	1976	1977	1978	1979	1980	1981	1982	1983	1984	1985	1986	1987	1988
Pneumonia	10	17	31	26	25	16	19	19	14	21	23	20	11
Septicaemia	0	2	6	8	10	7	9	9	9	17	12	18	14
NEC	1	2	4	7	3	4	6	2	6	4	2	4	5
Peritonitis*	4	1	9	4	4	1	4	0	1	4	0	7	3
Meningitis	1	2	6	2	5	0	3	1	1	2	3	1	0

NEC, necrotizing enterocolitis.
*Excludes NEC.

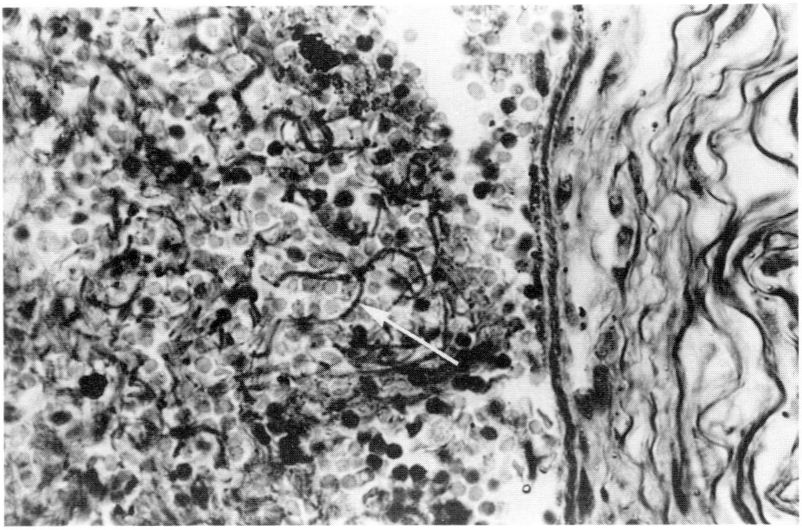

Fig. 2.3. Interlacing strands of fibrin (arrowed) inside a pulmonary vessel, the wall of which is on the right. (Stain: haematoxylin and eosin. Magnification: ×650.)

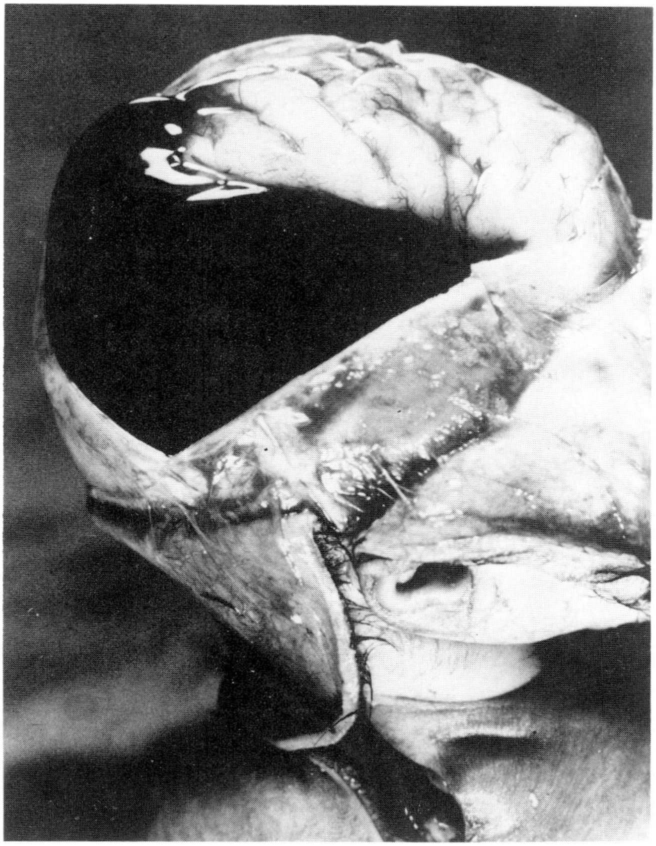

Fig. 2.4. A well-demarcated subarachnoid haematoma over the right parieto-occipital region of the cerebrum in a neonate.

Necrotizing enterocolitis

Forty-one infants had pathology typical of acute necrotizing enterocolitis (NEC) (Fig. 2.5). Intracardiac blood cultures were taken from 36 and peritoneal swabs from 14. Bacteria were grown from all the peritoneal swabs, but nine of the blood cultures were sterile (Table 2.9).

E. coli, coagulase-negative staphylococci, *Clostridium* sp. and streptococci were the most common pathogens. Out of the nine streptococcal isolates, five were non-haemolytic streptococci, with only a single isolate of group B streptococci.

The annual incidence of NEC varied between one and seven, with no overall trend (Table 2.8).

Nine infants with NEC had associated pathology which was thought to have an aetiological role. The most common of these was meconium ileus, which occurred in five. Intestinal obstruction secondary to Hirschsprung's disease, ileal atresia and diaphragmatic hernia were present in three other infants. An adverse reaction to indomethacin was thought to be a factor in another patient.

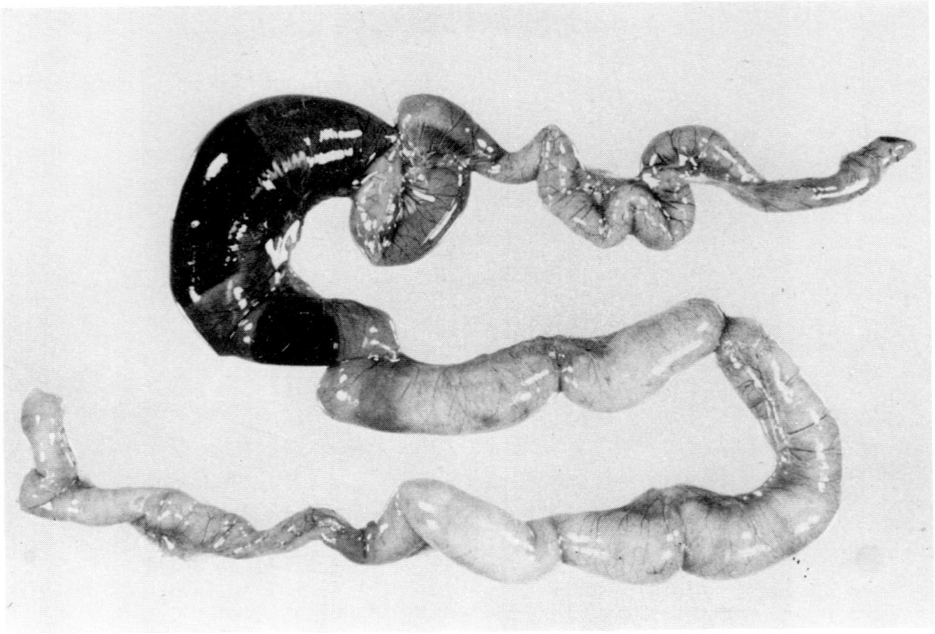

Fig. 2.5. Small intestine showing a well-defined haemorrhagic infarction associated with acute necrotizing enterocolitis.

Table 2.9. *Blood and peritoneal cultures from 50 infants dying with necrotizing enterocolitis*

Organism	Number of cases	
	Blood	Peritoneum
E. coli	11	6
Coagulase-negative staphylococci	6	6
Staph. aureus	0	1
Clostridium sp.	4	3
Pseudomonas sp.	2	4
Streptococcus sp.	6	3
Candida sp.	2	2
Enterobacter sp.	3	0
Proteus sp.	1	2
Klebsiella sp.	2	0
Haemophilus sp.	0	1
Citrobacter sp.	1	0
Acinetobacter sp.	0	1
Bacteroides sp.	1	0
No growth	9	0
Cases cultured	36	14

Peritonitis not due to necrotizing enterocolitis

Forty-two infants had a generalized peritonitis at necropsy but with neither pathological nor clinical evidence that it was secondary to acute NEC. Peritoneal exudate was cultured from 21 and blood cultures were collected from 22 (Table 2.10). The organisms isolated were similar to those found in the cases of NEC, with *E. coli*, *Clostridium* sp. and coagulase-negative staphylococci predominating.

The majority of these infants developed peritonitis secondary to anatomical obstruction of the intestine (Table 2.11). Thrombosis of the aorta and inferior vena cava from indwelling catheters had precipitated intestinal infarction in two. A peritoneal catheter had perforated the intestine in two others, following abdominal surgery. In nine infants the peritonitis was regarded as a

Table 2.10. *Blood and peritoneal cultures from 42 infants dying with peritonitis not secondary to necrotizing enterocolitis*

Organism	Number of cases	
	Blood	Peritoneum
E. coli	7	8
Coagulase-negative staphylococci	2	8
Clostridium sp.	2	5
Candida sp.	3	3
Pseudomonas sp.	1	3
Acinetobacter sp.	2	1
Enterobacter sp.	2	0
Proteus sp.	1	1
Citrobacter sp.	1	0
Enterococcus sp.	1	0
Group B streptococcus	1	0
Strep. faecalis	1	0
Bacteroides sp.	1	0
No growth	0	2
Cases cultured	22	21

complication of septicaemia originating elsewhere. In only two infants could no explanation be found. Although proof was lacking, there was suspicion that they had late complications of NEC.

Meningitis

Twenty-seven (3%) of the necropsies on liveborn infants gave histopathological evidence of meningitis, including one case of acute ventriculitis (Fig. 2.6). An additional infant had staphylococcal brain abscesses in the absence of meningeal inflammation.

Four infants had sterile CSF, despite morphological evidence of meningeal suppuration. In two of these, gram-positive coccobacilli were seen in histological sections of brain. Six infants had two or more organisms cultured from CSF *post mortem*. The bacteria identified are listed in Table 2.12. One infant had cerebral cytomegalovirus infection and five infants had cerebral candidiasis. *E. coli* and streptococcus were the most common bacteria isolated.

Table 2.11. *Underlying pathology in 42 infants dying with peritonitis not due to necrotizing enterocolitis*

Pathology	Number of cases
Septicaemia	9
Meconium ileus	5
Gastroschisis	4
Volvulus	4
Hirschsprung's disease	3
Rectal atresia	3
Duodenal atresia	2
Exomphalos	1
Hydrometrocolpos	1
Repaired diaphragmatic hernia	1
Malrotation	1
Gastric perforation	1
Inferior vena caval thrombosis	1
Aortic thrombosis	1
Intraperitoneal transfusion	1
Embolic infarction	1
Inguinal hernia	1
Unexplained	2

Table 2.12. *Organisms cultured from cerebrospinal fluid in 27 cases of fatal meningitis*

Organism		Number of cases
E. coli		6
Strep. viridans	2	6
Group B streptococcus	2	
Non-haemolytic streptococci	1	
Strep. pneumoniae	1	
Candida sp		5
Pseudomonas sp.		4
Staph. aureus	2	3
Coagulase-negative staphylococci	1	
Clostridium sp.		2
Acinetobacter sp.		1
Enterobacter sp.		1
Pneumococcus sp.		1
Proteus sp.		1
Bacteroides sp.		1
Cytomegalovirus		1
No growth		4
Total isolates		32

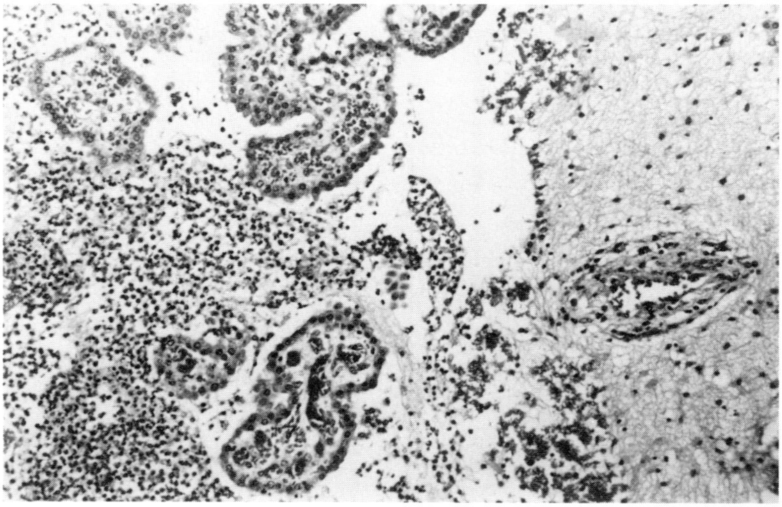

Fig. 2.6. Acute ventriculitis showing inflammatory exudate in the cavity of the lateral ventricle. Subependymal brain tissue is on the right. (Stain: haematoxylin and eosin. Magnification: ×150.)

Table 2.13. *Comparison of mean gestational age and survival time in different forms of fatal sepsis*

	Septi-caemia	NEC	Peritoni-tis*	Menin-gitis
Mean gestation (weeks)	32	33	35	31
Mean survival (days)	7	26	22	24
Total cases	121	50	42	27

NEC, necrotizing enterocolitis.
*Excludes NEC.

Relationship of infection to maturity and survival

The mean gestation age, as determined by dates, and the mean survival in postnatal days are set out in Table 2.4 for infants with bronchopneumonia and in Table 2.13 for those with septicaemia, NEC, peritonitis or meningitis.

The prematurity of all these groups merely reflects the high incidence of respiratory-distress syndrome, which was the most common reason for admission to the intensive care unit. The mean survival of the NEC, peritonitis and meningitis groups was in excess of 3 weeks, whereas most (58%) of the infants with bronchopneumonia were less than 1 week of age when they died. Infants dying with septicaemia had a mean age of 7 days and a gestational maturity similar to the other groups.

The relationship of some pathogens to survival times was striking. The group B streptococci and *Bacteroides fragilis* were probably derived from the birth canal and were associated with earlier deaths than were *Pseudomonas* sp. and *Candida* sp., which were more likely to be acquired on the intensive care unit (Table 2.14).

Non-bacterial pathogens in necropsies of liveborn infants

Of the infections other than bacteria, systemic candidiasis was by far the most common (Table 2.15). The lungs were the organ most

Table 2.14. *Relationship of four pathogens to survival among 383 liveborn infants dying from major infection*

Organism	Survival (days)			
	0–1	1–7	8–28	28+
Group B streptococcus	9	4	1	4
Bacteroides fragilis	2	5	1	0
Pseudomonas sp.	3	9	28	21
Candida sp.	0	0	9	24

Table 2.15. *Incidence of non-bacterial pathogens in 383 infants dying from infection and in 902 liveborn infants dying from all causes*

Pathogen	Number of necropsies	Percentage of infected necropsies	Percentage of all necropsies
Candida sp.	33	8.6	3.7
Cytomegalovirus	11	2.9	1.2
Other viruses	4	1.0	0.4
Mycoplasma sp.	1	0.3	0.1

Table 2.16. *Organ distribution of cytomegalovirus and Candida in necropsies*

Organ	Number of necropsies	
	Cytomegalovirus	Candida
Lung	10	24
Kidney	11	10
Brain	2	10
Heart	0	10
Intestine/peritoneum	1	8
Pancreas	7	1
Spleen	1	6
Liver	5	4
Adrenal	1	5
Thyroid	3	3
Bladder	0	2
Ovary	1	0
Thymus	0	1
Aorta	0	2
Pituitary	0	1
Marrow	0	1
Inferior vena cava	0	1
Total cases	13	33

often involved (Table 2.16). Candidal spores and hyphae were usually a component of a thrombus blocking small or medium-sized pulmonary vessels and associated with a necrotizing vasculitis (Fig. 2.7). Systemic candidiasis was a recently developed problem on the intensive care unit, 18 (55%) of the cases occurring in the last 4 years of the study.

Cytomegalic inclusions are easily identifiable in histological preparations of lung, kidney and pancreas (Fig. 2.8; Table 2.16). In addition to the two cases already described involving stillbirths, there were 11 cases involving deaths of liveborn infants. Eight of these were thought to have acquired cytomegalovirus postnatally from transfusions of unscreened blood. As a group they were essentially small babies who had had prolonged intensive care. Their mean body weight at death was 1055 g and their mean survival was 59 days. In this respect they were not dissimilar to the infants who had died with candidiasis: these had a mean weight of 1028 g and a mean survival of 37 days. There were three other deaths of liveborn infants who were considered on clinical grounds to have acquired cytomegalovirus *in utero*. These infants all weighed more than 2 kg, as did the stillbirths with cytomegalovirus infection. It is worth noting that during the period of the study, but not included in it, there were two domiciliary cot deaths of infants who had histological evidence of cytomegalovirus infection at necropsy.

Three other viral infections were recognized during the study, but only one was culture positive. Parvovirus B19 was cultured from the liver of an infant with non-rhesus hydrops who survived for 45 min. Characteristic inclusions and necrosis were seen histologically (Fig. 2.9). There was a case of

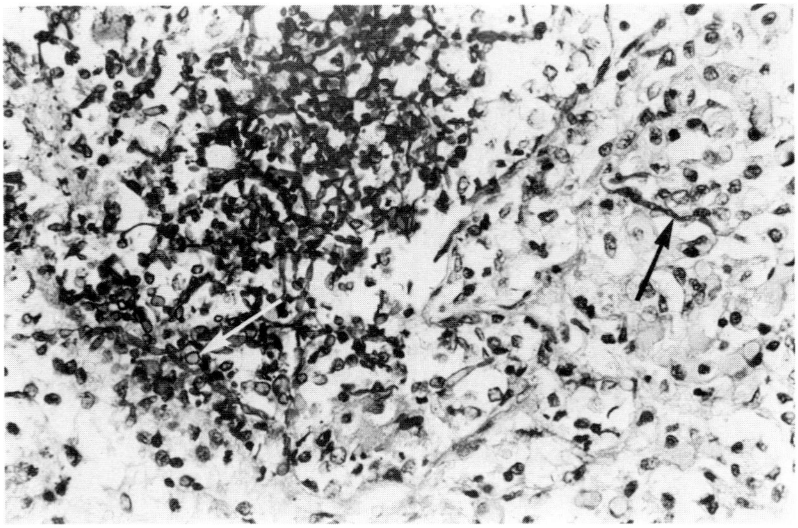

Fig. 2.7. Candidal spores (white arrow) blocking a small vessel and causing a vasculitis. Hyphae (black arrow) are invading adjacent tissue. (Stain: haematoxylin and eosin. Magnification: ×350.)

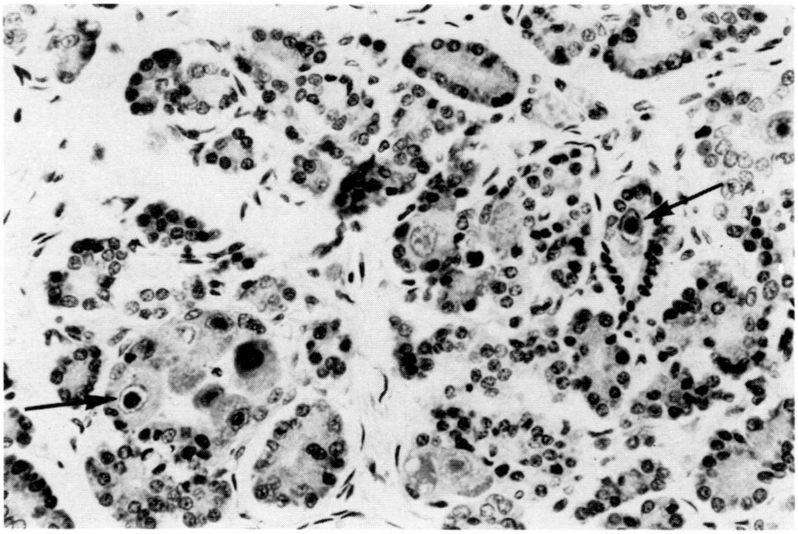

Fig. 2.8. Cytomegalic inclusions (arrowed) in pancreas. (Stain: haematoxylin and eosin. Magnification ×350.)

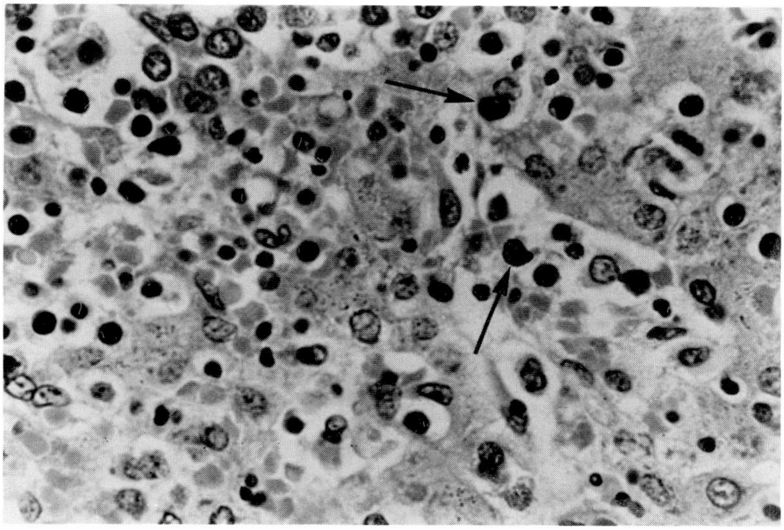

Fig. 2.9. Parvovirus inclusions (arrowed) in the liver of an infant with hydrops fetalis. (Stain: haematoxylin and eosin. Magnification: $\times 750$.)

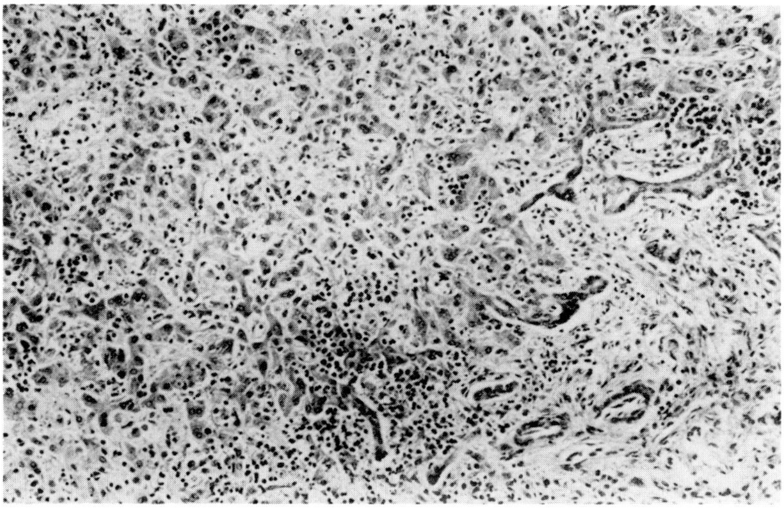

Fig. 2.10. Haemorrhagic infarction, inflammation and bile-duct proliferation in an infant who also had adrenal and renal necrosis. He was thought to have echovirus infection. (Stain: haematoxylin and eosin. Magnification: $\times 150$.)

congenital varicella in an infant whose mother had been infected at 20 weeks gestation. When the chronically sick infant died at 5 months, the infection had resolved, leaving focal calcification in the liver, kidney and spleen. A third infant had haemorrhagic infarction of the liver, adrenals and kidneys (Fig. 2.10). Although virological culture was negative, the histopathology was strongly suggestive of echovirus infection.

Mycoplasma, which strictly should be classified as a bacterial infection, occurred in one case. The infant died at 16 h, with bronchopneumonia and oesophagitis. The histopathology was not specific, but the organism was grown from lung tissue and in view of the short survival was probably intrauterine in origin.

Discussion

It is important to consider the role of infection in relationship to all the other causes of perinatal mortality. But the key word here is the word *causes*. The concept of a precise cause of death is something peculiar to the eye of the beholder. For any single death an obstetrician, a paediatrician and a pathologist will tend to cite different causes which reflect their personal involvement with the case (17). Thus a pathologist may attribute death to pneumonia which a paediatrician sees as essentially secondary to respiratory-distress syndrome in a premature birth, whilst an obstetrician will dismiss both these diagnoses as inevitable consequences of placental abruption. All in their own way are correct, but despite the inherent difficulty and bias of the exercise many previous surveys of the cause of perinatal deaths have adopted a system of specifying only what the author felt was the *primary* cause of death (9, 11, 13, 14). For example, in the British Perinatal Mortality Survey of 1958, pulmonary infection was seen by a panel of pathologists as the primary cause of death in 4.8% of the perinatal deaths, 13.3% of the early neonatal and 25.8% of the late neonatal deaths (9).

An approach which lends itself more to interdisciplinary agreement is to place perinatal deaths in broad categories. Thus, of 440 perinatal deaths in St Mary's Hospital between 1976 and 1981, 127 were macerated stillbirths without malformation, 109 were attributed to lethal malformation, 107 to the consequences of immaturity, 72 to birth asphyxia or trauma, and 25 to certain specific conditions (18). Within these categories infection played an increasingly important role during this period among the immature deaths and a consistently minor role in the macerated and asphyxial groups. In any retrospective review of perinatal and neonatal deaths it is more important to know the broad characteristics of the patients under study and the incidence of particular diseases within them than to have a personal opinion on what are considered to be the primary causes of death.

The present survey defines the incidence of infection at necropsy solely on histopathological observation, supported and clarified by bacteriological culture, without making any judgement on its relative influence with other concurrent pathology in causing death. The only opinion I am personally prepared to venture is that, where an infection is sufficiently established to provoke an inflammatory cellular response in vital internal organs, it would be imprudent to maintain that the infection was not at least one factor in the patient's death. The current technological sophistication of intensive care applied to ever-more premature infants has simultaneously created iatrogenic pathology (19) and prolonged survival. Neonatal death is now more multifactorial than it has ever been. In such circumstances it is a more objective and helpful exercise to assess the incidence of infection than to debate the nuances of its contribution to mortality.

In comparison with infection in liveborn infants, intrauterine infection is relatively infrequent. However, there is evidence that it has not always been so. Langley reviewed 275 stillbirths in St Mary's Hospital in the early 1950s (20) and found histological pneumonia in 28 (10%). This was compared with an incidence of 31% in a previously published Finnish study. In the current survey, pneumonia in stillbirths was found to occur in 1.1%, a tenth of what it was 20–30 years previously in the same hospital. There were two stillbirths with listeriosis. Apart from occasional outbreaks from infected milk (21) and a higher prevalence in northern France, clinically recognized cases are rare, even though the carrier rate in the human population is 5%. Treatment in liveborn infants can be successful, but most cases are only diagnosed after intrauterine death (22). The two cases of listeriosis reported here were among seven diagnosed over a 12-month period in St Mary's Hospital (23). Three cases survived after treatment and two are not included because they were aborted before 28 weeks gestation. The diagnosis is far more likely to be made in laboratories which culture specifically for *Listeria* sp. Only one of the mothers involved had had an influenza-like illness.

Cytomegalovirus infection is reported to have an incidence of 0.4–2.3% among liveborn infants in the USA (24). Of these, 5–10% may be anticipated to have symptoms at birth and 20% of them will die. There were five cases of intrauterine cytomegalovirus infection in the present study, two of whom were stillborn, representing a natural incidence (as opposed to an iatrogenic, or postnatally acquired, incidence) of 0.009% of births. This probably reflects a different geographical distribution of the virus.

Among the deaths in liveborn infants the dominant infection was pneumonia, occurring in nearly 28% of cases. Doubtless this is a secondary consequence of the respiratory difficulties accompanying prematurity, which overshadow neonatal mortality figures. Even before the establishment of intensive care units, pneumonia accounted for more than a quarter of the late-neonatal deaths in the British Perinatal Mortality Survey (9). Similar but smaller studies in the USA at about the same time put the incidence of pneumonia in the newborn at 24% (25) and 33% (26).

In the pneumonic group dying on the first postnatal day, histological examination of the placenta was performed in 13 infants, all but one of whom had evidence of an acute chorioamnionitis, often accompanied by acute funiculitis (Fig. 2.11). Three out of four stillbirths with pneumonia also had chorioamnionitis. However, the incidence of inflammation of the amnion and the cord is far in excess of the incidence of pneumonia. In a study of 1000 placentas in St Mary's Hospital (27), polymorphonuclear leucocyte infiltration of the placenta was seen in 24% and in the umbilical cord in 7%. A more recent study in a smaller series in Birmingham (28) put the incidence at 49% and 10% respectively.

In both studies a relationship to prolonged rupture of the membranes was observed, although how often infection preceded rather than followed such rupture is not clear. The assumption must be that only in a small minority of these cases was intrauterine pneumonia a complication. It is possible also that some cases of immediately postnatal pneumonia are derived not from aspiration of infected liquor but from bacteria lining the birth canal.

Although bacteriological culture is essential for the identification of the pathogen, there are two forms of pneumonia where the histopathology is very characteristic of the infecting organism. *Pseudomonas* bronchopneumonia typically leads to foci of necrosis and haemorrhage which are very distinctive (Fig. 2.12). On high magnification, gram-negative rods may be seen adhering to the

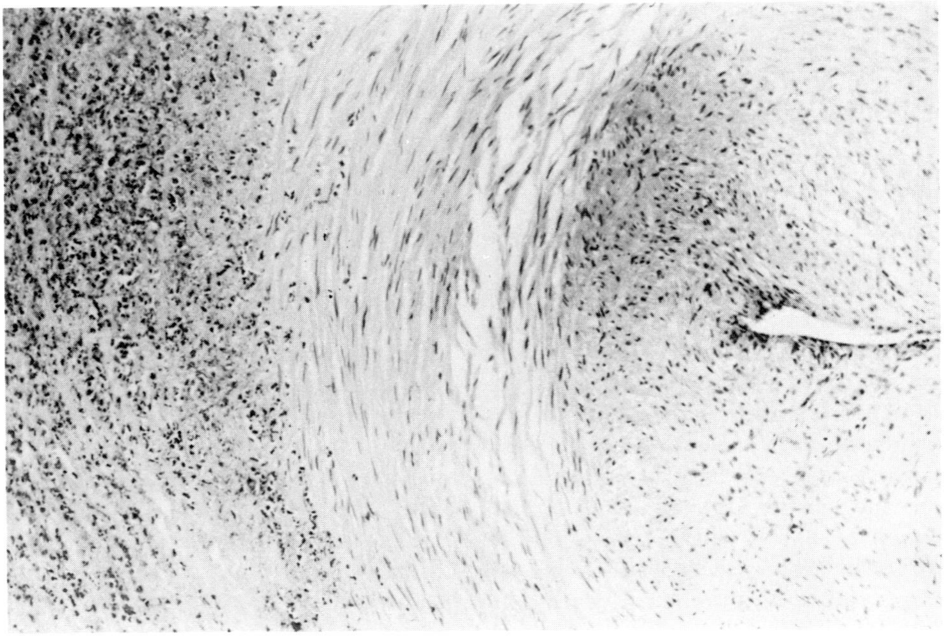

Fig. 2.11. An umbilical artery on the right with an acute inflammation of Wharton's jelly on the left. (Stain: haematoxylin and eosin. Magnification: ×150.)

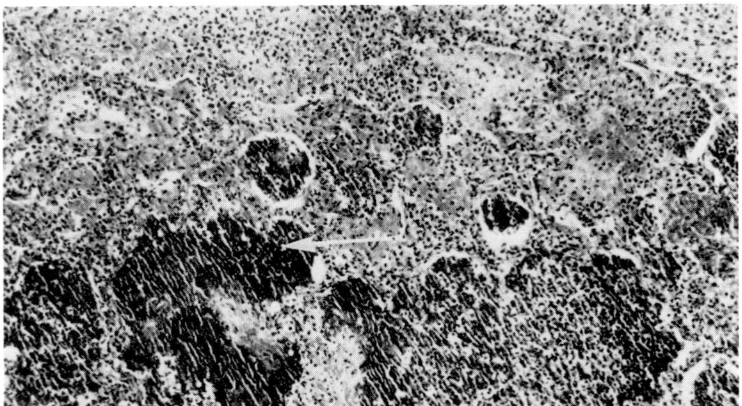

Fig. 2.12. Intense focal necrosis (arrowed) and haemorrhage in the lung of an infant with pseudomonal bronchopneumonia. (Stain: haematoxylin and eosin. Magnification: ×150.)

walls of small vessels without inducing intravascular thrombosis or any marked white cell response. *Pseudomonas* sp. thrives in moist conditions, and colonization of humidified ventilatory apparatus is a very real hazard of the intensive care unit (29).

A second form of bacterial pneumonia with a characteristic histopathological appearance is caused by group B streptococcus, which has an affinity for colonizing hyaline membranes (30, 31). So dense is this colonization that the normally pink eosinophilic hyaline membranes assume a blue colour. (Fig. 2.13). A rising incidence of group B streptococcus has caused concern at some centres (32–34), whilst an increase in staphylococcal infections has been a greater problem elsewhere (4, 5). However, as a cause of both bronchopneumonia and septicaemia, *E. coli* predominated in the present study, as it does in other hospitals (15, 35).

Neonatal septicaemia has increased significantly in intensive care units with increased survival (4). It is more common in infants referred from outside units (5), and in the majority of cases it is a terminal complication of already established sepsis rather than a primary cause of death (35). In the present study it was apparent that septicaemia in the necropsy population had increased in frequency over the decade in a way which could not be demonstrated for other forms of sepsis such as meningitis, peritonitis and NEC (Table 2.8).

These last three conditions accounted for 31% of the infected infants seen at necropsy in comparison with septicaemia (32%) and pneumonia (66%) (Table 2.3). The commonest pathogen was *E. coli*, although with meningitis there were an equal number of cases due to various streptococci. The majority of infants with meningitis, peritonitis or NEC also had positive blood cultures.

Most of the pneumonic deaths occurred at under 2 weeks of age, but infants with other infections survived longer (Tables 2.4 and 2.13). Since hyaline membrane disease predominates in the first 2 weeks and bronchopulmonary dysplasia in the latter half of the first month (Table 2.4), it might be

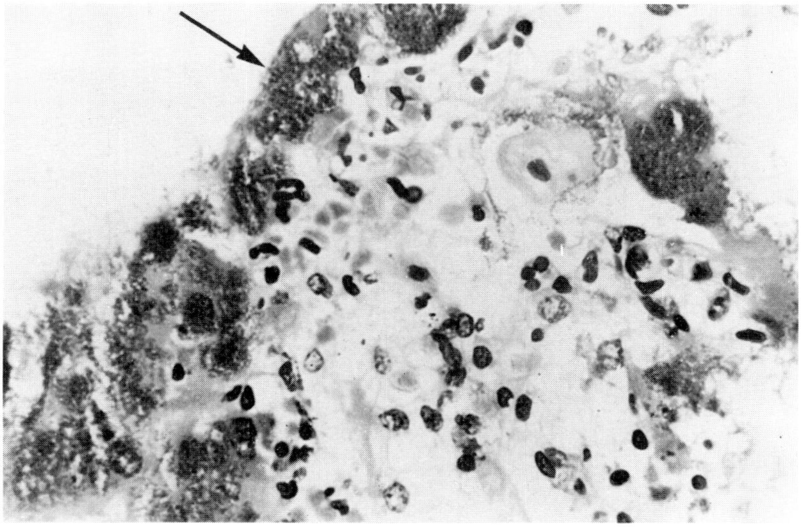

Fig. 2.13. Dense colonization of a hyaline membrane (arrowed) by cocci in an infant infected with haemolytic group B streptococci. (Stain: haematoxylin and eosin. Magnification: ×650.)

concluded that respiratory difficulty from lack of surfactant predisposes to infection more than the pathological effects of excess oxygen. However, this may be an erroneous conclusion, because selection of referrals to the unit may have biased the consequences.

Infection in this study has not been related to the incidence of intrauterine growth retardation. It has been shown previously (36) that intrauterine infection is no commoner in light-for-dates infants, presumably because it is largely acquired just before or during delivery. On the other hand, pulmonary infections were found more frequently in these infants, especially after the third postnatal day.

The iatrogenic aspects of infection on the neonatal intensive care unit cannot be overemphasized. The three initial hurdles for the premature infant who is without congenital malformation are birth asphyxia, hyaline membrane disease and intraventricular haemorrhage, often in that sequence. The risk of pneumonia is directly related to the duration of ventilation. Umbilical arterial catheterization commonly induces aortic thrombus formation. The thrombus may then become infected via the catheter and act as a nidus for the systemic dissemination of bacteria (Fig. 2.14). A mycotic aortic aneurysm arose by this means in one infant in the series and five others have been reported in the literature since 1976 (37). In recent years, long central venous lines have found favour for the chronically sick newborn infant. Unfortunately, such catheters carry an appreciable risk of systemic candidiasis (38). Parenteral lipid infusion and multiple courses of antibiotics to treat repeated episodes of pneumonia are also potent risk factors for candidiasis (39).

The sharp rise in deaths with systemic candidiasis seen in the present survey is a reflection of the increasing proportion of infants of very low birthweight being treated on the intensive care unit. Infants weighing under 1 kg are particularly susceptible to fungal colonization (40). The combination of broad-spectrum chemotherapy with parenteral feeding often leads to intestinal colonization by *Candida* sp. The gut then provides a reservoir for infection spreading systemically either directly via NEC and perforation or, more commonly, by contamination of

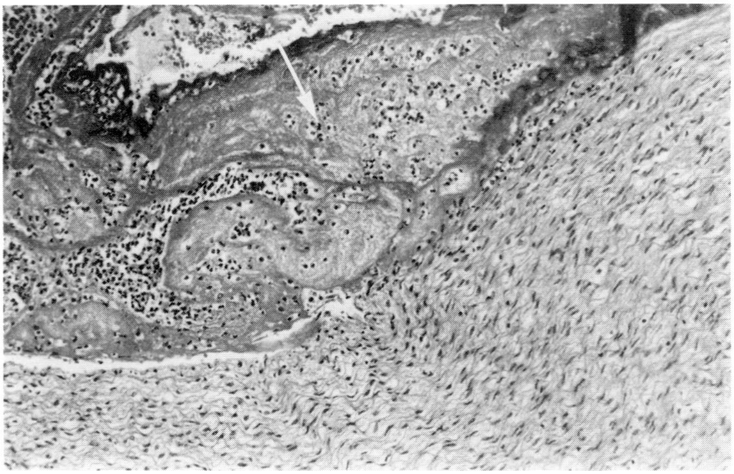

Fig. 2.14. Acute inflammatory cells (arrowed) within a thrombus adherent to the wall of the aorta on the lower right of the figure. (Stain: haematoxylin and eosin. Magnification: ×150.)

catheters or endotracheal tubes. Medical and nursing personnel should be aware not only that infants of very low birthweight are immunologically immature but also that the physical distance between the anus and a endotracheal tube is very much less than is the case with an adult.

Only five of the 13 cases of systemic cytomegalovirus infection in the survey were thought to have been acquired naturally. Eight cases were induced by transfusions with unscreened blood. The risks involved by this practice have been well documented (41). However, the use of seronegative donor blood is not without some danger, since such donors may have been recently infected (42)

Cytomegalic inclusions are relatively easy for the histopathologist to recognize. Other viral inclusions are more subtle in their morphology, and routine virological culture of all necropsies puts an unrewarding burden on the laboratory. There is a strong case for routinely culturing for parvovirus in all infants with non-rhesus hydrops who are devoid of any gross anatomical explanation for the oedema. The light microscopic features and electron microscopy are characteristic (43). The massive hepatic necrosis seen with echovirus 11 associated with adrenal haemorrhage and often following maternal gastroenteritis (44) requires culture to be certain of the diagnosis. Other viral infections which should be sought in the fetus and newborn are coxsackievirus B, varicella zoster and herpes simplex (45).

References

1. Hurley R, de Louvois J, Drasar F (eds). Perinatal and neonatal infections. J Antimicrob Chem 1979; 5 (Suppl A): 1–89.
2. Siegel JD, McCracken GH. Sepsis neonatorum. N Engl J Med 1981; 304: 642–7.
3. Rudel P, Peckham C. Infection of the fetus and the newborn: prevention, treatment and related handicap. Clin Obstet Gynecol 1988; 8: 55–71.
4. Bennet R, Eriksson M, Zelterstrom R. Increasing incidence of neonatal septicaemia: causative organism and predisposing risk factors. Acta Paediatr 1981; 70: 207–10.
5. Oro A. Major bacterial infection in a referral intensive care unit. J Infect 1982; 5: 117–26.
6. Hensey OJ, Hart CA, Cooke RWI. Serious infection in a neonatal intensive care unit: a two-year survey. J Hyg 1985; 95: 289–97.
7. Gau G. Is the perinatal necropsy really necessary? Arch Dis Child 1983; 58: 649–50.
8. Porter HJ, Keeling JW. Value of perinatal necropsy examination. J Clin Pathol 1987; 40: 180–4.
9. Butler NR, Bonham DG. Perinatal mortality: the first report of the 1958 British Perinatal Mortality Survey. Edinburgh: Churchill Livingstone, 1963.
10. Claireaux A. Stillbirths and first week deaths. In: British births, vol 1. London: Heinemann, 1970: 235–53.
11. Atwood HD, Stewart AD. Perinatal mortality: a clinicopathological study of 2000 necropsies. Aust NZ J Obstet Gynaecol 1968; 8: 33–41.
12. Valdes-Dapena MA, Arey JB. The causes of neonatal mortality: an analysis of 501 autopsies on newborn infants. J Pediatr 1970; 77: 366–75.
13. Machin GA. A perinatal mortality survey in south-east London, 1970–73: the pathological findings in 726 necropsies. J Clin Pathol 1975; 28: 428–34.
14. Joshi VV. Primary causes of perinatal mortality: autopsy study of 100 cases. Arch Pathol Lab Med 1976; 100: 106–9.
15. Pryse-Davies J, Hurley R. Infections and perinatal mortality. J Antimicrob Chemother 1979; 5 (A): 59–70.
16. Ohlsson A, Shennan AT, Rose TH. Review of causes of perinatal mortality in a regional perinatal center, 1980 to 1984. Am J Obstet Gynecol 1987; 157: 443–5.
17. Barson AJ. The contribution of pathology to perinatal audit. In: Chalmers I, McIlwaine G (eds) Perinatal audit and surveillance. London: Royal College of Obstetricians and Gynaecologists, 1980: 228–38.
18. Barson AJ, Tasker M, Lieberman BA, Hillier VF. Impact of improved perinatal care on the causes of death. Arch Dis Child 1984; 59: 199–207.
19. Keeling JW. Iatrogenic disease in the newborn. Virchows Arch [A] 1981; 394: 1–29.
20. Langley FA, McCredie-Smith JA. Perinatal pneumonia: a retrospective study. J Obstet Gynaecol 1959; 66: 12–25.

21. Barza M. Listeriosis and milk. N Engl J Med 1985; 312: 438–40.
22. Khong TY, Frappell JM, Steel HM, Stewart CM, Burke M. Perinatal listeriosis: a report of six cases. Br J Obstet Gynaecol 1986; 96: 1083–7.
23. Smith ARB, Lieberman BA, Allen L, Barson AJ. Listeriosis and pregnancy. Lancet 1983; 2: 1634.
24. Stagno S, Pass RF, Dworsky ME, Alford CA. Maternal cytomegalovirus infection and perinatal transmission. Clin Obstet Gynecol 1982; 25: 563–76.
25. Briggs NJ, Hogg G. Perinatal pulmonary pathology. Pediatrics 1958; 22: 41–8.
26. Landing BH. Pulmonary lesions in newborn infants: a statistical study. Pediatrics 1957; 19: 217–23.
27. Fox H, Langley FA. Leukocyte infiltration of the placenta and umbilical cord: a clinico-pathology study. Obstet Gynecol 1971; 37: 451–8.
28. Chellam VG, Rushton DI. Chorioamnionitis and funiculitis in placentas of 200 births weighing less than 2.5 kg. Br J Obstet Gynaecol 1985; 92: 808–814.
29. Barson AJ. Fatal *Pseudomonas aeruginosa* bronchopneumonia in a children's hospital. Arch Dis Child 1971; 46: 55–60.
30. Ablow RC, Driscoll SG, Effman EL, Gross I, Jolles CJ, Uauy R, Warshaw JB. A comparison of early-onset group B streptococcal neonatal infection and the respiratory-distress syndrome of the newborn. N Engl J Med 1976; 294: 65–70.
31. Katzenstein A, Davis C, Braude A. Pulmonary changes in neonatal sepsis due to group B beta-hemolytic streptococcus: relation to hyaline membrane disease. J Infect Dis 1976; 133: 430–5.
32. Freedman RM, Ingram DL, Gross I, Ehrenkranz RA, Warshaw B, Baltimore RS. A half century of neonatal sepsis at Yale, 1928 to 1978. Am J Dis Child 1981; 135: 140–4.
33. Pass MA, Gray BM, Khare S, Dillon HC Jr. Prospective studies of group B streptococcal infections in infants. J Pediatr 179; 95: 437–43.
34. Editorial. Neonatal infection with group B streptococci. Lancet 1981; 2: 181–2.
35. Hurley R, de Louvois J. Bloodstream infections and perinatal mortality. J Clin Pathol 1981; 34: 271–6.
36. Fedrick J. Neonatal deaths: time of death, maturity and lesions. Biol Neonate 1971; 18: 369–78.
37. Colclough AB, Barson AJ, Infantile aortic aneurysm complicating umbilical arterial catheterisation. Arch Dis Child 1981; 56: 795–7.
38. Grisoni ER, Mehta SK, Connors AF. Thrombosis and infection complicating central venous catheterisation in neonates. J Pediatr Surg 1986; 21: 772–6.
39. Knox WF, Hooton VN, Barson AJ. Pulmonary vascular candidiasis and use of central venous catheters in neonates. J Clin Pathol 1987; 40: 559–65.
40. Baley JE, Kliegman RM, Boxerbaum B, Fanaroff AA. Fungal colonisation in very low birth weight infants. Pediatrics 1986; 78: 225–32.
41. Yeager AS, Grumet FC, Hafleigh EB, Aroni AM, Bradley JS. Prober CG. Prevention of transfusion-acquried cytomegalovirus infections in newborn infants. J Pediatr 1981; 98: 281–7.
42. Logan S, Barbara J, Kovar. I Cytomegalovirus screened blood for neonatal intensive care units. Arch Dis Child 1988; 63: 753–5.
43. Knisely AS, O'Shea PA, McMillan P, Singer DB, Magid MS. Electron microscopic identification of parvovirus virions in erythroid-line cells in fatal hydrops fetalis. Ped Pathol 1988; 8: 163–70.
44. Mostoufizadeh M, Lack EE, Gang DL, Perez-Atayde AR, Driscoll SG. Postmortem manifestations of echovirus 11 sepsis in five newborn infants. Hum Pathol 1983; 14: 818–23.
45. Benirsche K, Robb JA. Infectious causes of fetal death. Clin Obstet Gynecol 1987; 30: 284–94.

3 Hospital-Acquired Infections

D. Isaacs
John Radcliffe Hospital, Oxford, UK

Definition

The term *nosocomial*, from the Greek word for hospital, literally means 'of or related to hospital'. For the newborn, it has come conventionally to be used to describe hospital-acquired as opposed to perinatally acquired infections. As a rule hospital-acquired infections will tend to be of relatively late onset, whereas perinatally acquired infections will present early, in the first week and often in the first 48 h after birth. Babies may, however, become colonized with organisms acquired from the maternal genital tract at birth and these organisms may later invade and cause infection; such infection is vertically acquired and has been termed *auto-infection* as opposed to nosocomial infection (1). Unless cultures are taken from all babies at birth, it may be impossible to determine whether maternal or hospital-acquired organisms are responsible for late-onset sepsis, yet the distinction is important since nosocomial infections are potentially preventable. Iatrogenic infections are 'caused by doctors' and some nosocomial infections are iatrogenic, although these are to an extent an inevitable concomitant of the neonatal intensive care environment.

Incidence and outcome

The reported incidence of nosocomial infections in nurseries depends on the definition of sepsis, the level of intensive care, the intensity of surveillance of infections and many other factors. Nosocomial infection rates as low as 0.6% of babies in community hospitals in the USA and as high as 30% of babies admitted to a Dutch newborn intensive care unit (1) have been described.

The outcome of hospital-acquired infections is generally more favourable than that of perinatally acquired infections. In Oxford, over 3 years from 1984 to 1987, there were only two deaths from 45 episodes of late-onset (after 48 h) hospital-acquired septicaemia or meningitis, but 10 deaths from 27 episodes of early-onset (first 48 h after birth) vertically acquired infections. Hoogkamp-Korstanje et al. reported that three out of nine babies with nosocomial infections due to *Pseudomonas aeruginosa* died, but 46 babies infected with other organisms all survived, suggesting that *Ps. aeruginosa* may be more virulent (1).

The incidence of late-onset sepsis is greatest in babies of very low birthweight. In Oxford, babies of birthweight 1500–2499 g have the same rate of sepsis after the first 48 h of life as babies of birthweight 2500 g and over admitted to the neonatal unit – 0.8% of both groups become infected. More than 10% of babies of 1000–1499 g and more than 20% of babies under 1000 g, however, developed late-onset infections (Table 3.1).

Infection in the Newborn. Edited by J. de Louvois and D. Harvey
©1990 John Wiley & Sons Ltd

Table 3.1. *Late-onset sepsis: bacteraemia or meningitis after 48 h of age (NICU, John Radcliffe Hospital, Oxford; 1.5.84–31.10.85)*

Birthweight (g)	Sepsis	Total	Proportion infected
<2500	3	371	0.8%
1500–2499	2	266	0.8%
1000–1499	11	95	11.6%
<1000	11	54	20.4%
All babies	27	786	3.4%

NICU, neonatal intensive care unit.

Table 3.2. *Risk factors associated with nosocomial infections in neonates stratified for birthweight (Boston Children's Hospital 1974–1977)*

	Relative risk	95% confidence intervals	*P*
Endotracheal intubation	7.0	1.8–25.1	<0.01
Hyperalimentation	5.9	1.9–21.8	<0.01
Patent ductus arteriosus	28.2	3.7–21.3	<0.001

From Goldmann et al. (2).

Factors affecting incidence of sepsis

Preterm and even term neonates are immunologically immature and are subjected to invasive procedures and to a wide range of potential pathogens in the intensive care environment.

Goldmann et al. have examined the risk factors for nosocomial infections in babies admitted to their nursery for the newborn (2). Many of the factors were interrelated and the authors did not perform a multivariate analysis, although they did stratify for birthweight since the incidence of infections was inversely related to birthweight. The three factors found to be significantly associated with the development of nosocomial infection were endotracheal intubation, hyperalimentation and patent ductus arteriosus (Table 3.2). Endotracheal intubation predisposes to pneumonia, but is only done in the sicker babies; interestingly, respiratory-distress syndrome was only associated with a relative risk of sepsis of 1.2 (95% confidence intervals 0.4–3.9). Hyperalimentation also identified sick babies; the siting of silastic intravenous cannulas ('central lines'), which may become colonized with organisms such as *Staphylococcus epidermidis*, may contribute to risk of infection. Patent ductus arteriosus was often associated with prolonged ventilation and hyperalimentation.

Patient-to-staff ratios or workload have been linked to the incidence of infections. The risk of nosocomial infection fell from 5.2% of infants in a crowded, hectic newborn nursery to 0.9% when the nursery moved to a new site with 50% more nurses, increased space per infant, convenient sinks and isolation facilities (2). This was a sequential study, but the patient population was essentially unchanged and the difference in incidence of infection was statistically highly significant. Overcrowding has also been implicated in outbreaks of infection with *Staphylococcus aureus* (3). Using a scoring system weighted for level of intensive care, it has been shown that the incidence of colonization with gentamicin-resistant gram-negative organisms is strongly associated with workload (4).

Umbilical catheters are commonly used in neonatal care. Umbilical arterial catheters rarely become infected (5), whereas umbilical venous catheters (UVCs) often become colonized and may cause septicaemia. The frequency of colonization of UVCs is the same in babies who do or do not receive antibiotics and does not depend on duration of catheterization or the type of local preparation used on the umbilicus (6–8).

Any break in the infant's skin predisposes to local and thence systemic sepsis. Scalp electrodes, particularly spiral electrodes, have

Table 3.3. *Organisms isolated from infections resulting from the use of scalp electrodes*

Herpes simplex virus
Haemophilus influenzae
Group A streptococcus
Group B streptococcus
Neisseria gonorrhoeae
Anaerobic bacteria

Scalp abscess, osteomyelitis and disseminated herpes simplex have been described as complications arising out of use of scalp electrodes, particularly spiral electrodes.

caused local abscesses due to a number of different organisms from the maternal genital tract (Table 3.3). Bacteraemia and osteomyelitis of the skull have been described as complications, as has disseminated herpes simplex virus (HSV) infection (9). The use of electrocardiograph electrodes which penetrated the skin was associated with local abscesses. The site of entry of peripheral and central catheters may become infected, as more rarely may chest drains and other invasive devices. Even relatively innocuous interventions such as urine bags may cause breakdown of the thin skin of preterm infants and lead to infection.

The overuse of antibiotics, as will be discussed later, may cause the emergence of resistant organisms and predispose to candidaemia. But, in addition, it may alter the normal flora and predispose to colonization with potentially pathogenic bacteria. Goldmann et al. found that babies given more than 3 days of antibiotics were significantly more likely than babies given 3 or less days to develop nasopharyngeal colonization with gram-negative bacteria (43% vs 19%) and bowel colonization with *Klebsiella* spp., *Enterobacter* spp. and *Citrobacter* spp. (10).

Modes of transmission of infection

Infection develops at a variable time following colonization with organisms, or from direct inoculation. Various modes of transmission of infection with different organisms are shown in Table 3.4. The single most commonly implicated mode of transmission is via the hands of staff, and this may in turn be more likely to occur in overcrowded nurseries with high patient-to-staff ratios.

Organisms causing nosocomial infection

Gram-negative bacilli

In the 1970s widespread colonization with gram-negative enteric organisms was described in nurseries for the newborn, particularly in developed countries. Organisms such as *Escherichia coli*, *Klebsiella* spp., *Pseudomonas* spp., *Serratia* spp. and other bacilli, which rarely caused septicaemia except in immunocompromised patients, became responsible for an increasing proportion of episodes of bacteraemia, meningitis and other infections, such as pneumonia and skin sepsis. A similar increase in incidence in adult cases was simultaneously described (11). In the early 1960s most *E. coli* were susceptible to ampicillin, but plasmid-mediated beta-lactamase resistance rapidly emerged and over half of all hospital-acquired *E. coli* are now ampicillin resistant. Plasmid-mediated resistance to aminoglycosides has also developed, and although there is some evidence that aminoglycoside-resistant gram-negative bacteria may sometimes be less virulent than sensitive ones (12, 13), nevertheless several outbreaks of disease due to resistant organisms have been described (see table 29-1 in reference 5).

Gastrointestinal colonization of neonates is an important reservoir of infection; organisms may be carried for prolonged periods on the hands of staff (14) and transmitted between infants. Nasojejunal tube-feeding rapidly leads to abnormal colonization of the jejunum with coliform bacilli (15). Many of the

Table 3.4. *Modes of transmission of infection*

Gram-negative enteric bacteria	Hands of staff (overcrowding) Resuscitation equipment Eyewash Scrubbing brushes
Staphylococcus aureus	Hands of staff (overcrowding) Baby's skin
Coagulase-negative staphylococci	Hands of staff Baby's skin
Enterobacter spp.	Contaminated intravenous fluids
Listeria monocytogenes	Rectal thermometer Delivery suite
Respiratory syncytial virus	Hands of staff Staff infections
Enteroviruses (echo, coxsackie)	Hands of staff Staff infections
Rhizopus	Surgical bandages

gram-negative enteric organisms can thrive in water, and water has in the past been a source of infection. Resuscitation equipment has caused transmission of *Ps. aeruginosa* and eyewash solutions have caused two outbreaks of infection with coliforms (5), but the hands of nursery staff are the most commonly suspected or proven mode of transmission. *Pseudomonas* spp. may commonly be found on taps and in sinks, but when careful typing is done the patients are generally found to become colonized with other pseudomonads from mothers, staff or other babies (16). Outbreaks of infection with *Enterobacter* spp. have been caused by contaminated intravenous (IV) fluids.

In Oxford, gram-negative bacteria together form the largest group of organisms causing septicaemia or meningitis after 48 h of age (Table 3.5).

Table 3.5. *Organisms causing late-onset systemic sepsis (after 48 h of age) (NICU, John Radcliffe Hospital, Oxford; 1.5.84–30.4.87)*

Organism	Number of isolates
Enterococci	15
Pseudomonas spp.	12
Klebsiella spp.	9
Staphylococcus epidermidis	9
Escherichia coli	6
Other gram-negative organisms	6
Staphylococcus aureus	1
Clostridium sp.	1
Total	59

45 episodes, 13 polymicrobial.

NICU, neonatal intensive care unit.

Enterococci

Enterococci are increasingly being recognized as causes of nosocomial infection in nurseries for the newborn; in Oxford they currently outnumber any other single organism (Table 3.5). There are no specific features of infection and, although the mortality is lower than with gram-negative organisms such as *Pseudomonas* spp., meningitis may occur. Enterococci are resistant to the newer cephalosporins, providing a strong argument against their routine use, at least alone, in 'blind' treatment of late-onset sepsis in nurseries where enterococci are prevalent.

Staphylococcus aureus

Staphylococcus aureus was responsible for epidemics of sepsis in the USA and UK in the 1950s and 1960s, and the use of flucloxacillin with an aminoglycoside to treat late-onset sepsis in many British nurseries is partly based on this. With improved skin and cord care such epidemics are now rare. Occasional outbreaks of bullous impetigo may now be seen as a warning that infection-control measures have become lax. Methicillin-resistant *Staph. aureus* strains appeared in the late 1960s and, perhaps following widespread use of gentamicin, re-emerged in the late 1970s. The genes coding for methicillin resistance are usually chromosomal, not plasmid-borne, rendering the resistance more stable. Resistance to antiseptics such as chlorhexidine also occurs (17). Colonization is far more common than systemic sepsis, but cases and indeed epidemics of sepsis have occurred, in which case vancomycin is the treatment of choice.

Staphylococcus epidermidis

Coagulase-negative staphylococci, particularly *Staph. epidermidis* are skin commensals and common contaminants of blood and cerebrospinal fluid (CSF) cultures. They are also adept at colonizing synthetic materials such as silastic intravascular cannulas and CSF shunts, and an important determinant is thought to be the ability of some strains to secrete a glycocalyx or slime layer in which colonies can grow and be protected from host defence mechanisms and antibiotics. Hall et al. found that colonizing staphylococci from infants with coagulase-negative staphylococcal septicaemia were more likely to be slime producers than were organisms from colonized infants without sepsis (18).

Reports of an increasing incidence of coagulase-negative staphylococcal infections should be read with a certain scepticism since many papers do not distinguish contaminated blood cultures from true sepsis. There is no doubt that these organisms can cause severe sepsis however, and in recent reports from the UK (19) and from Holland (1) they were responsible for a third to a half of all nosocomial infections. In Oxford, where central lines are rarely used and enteral feeding is commenced very early in most babies, *Staph. epidermidis* sepsis is rarer, albeit increasing in frequency. Although central lines are a definite risk factor, the organisms may also be carried on the hands of staff (1) and have been described as contaminants in IV fluids (20). *Staph. epidermidis* is being recognized as an important cause of pneumonia, 14 out of 29 patients with coagulase-negative staphylococcal bacteraemia in one study having new or increasing pulmonary infiltrates (18).

Kirpalani et al. found serum C-reactive protein measurements and immature to total white cell counts useful in addition to clinical data in attempting to distinguish true episodes of coagulase-negative staphylococcal septicaemia from contaminated blood cultures (21).

Cultures drawn through central lines may only reflect colonization and septicaemia should be confirmed by peripheral venous cultures. Infected central lines usually need to be removed while infected shunts can rarely be sterilized with antibiotics alone.

The incidence of isolates resistant to multiple antibiotics including methicillin has been increasing and in some parts of the UK these are the leading cause of late-onset sepsis, necessitating the use of vancomycin as first-line treatment for suspected late-onset sepsis.

Group B streptococcus

About 8% of infants born to mothers whose cultures are negative for group B streptococcus at delivery become colonized with the organism within 48 h. Nosocomial colonization is most likely when there is a high prevalence and when there is overcrowding and poor hand-washing (22–24). There is a very low attack rate for disease in infants nosocomially colonized, since they are generally less heavily colonized than babies with vertical transmission and sepsis depends largely on the microbial load (25). Infants colonized or infected with group B streptococci do not, therefore, need to be isolated.

Fungi

The incidence of systemic fungal infections appears to be increasing, and although the great majority of infections are caused by *Candida albicans*, there have also been reports of wound infections with *Rhizopus*, which has contaminated surgical bandages (26), and an unexplained outbreak of systemic infection with *Hansenula anomala* in Liverpool (27). *Candida* is ubiquitous and commonly causes mucosal and skin infections. Abscesses may develop with systemic infection, and pus should always be examined using Gram's stain. Systemic infection occurs particularly in babies of very low birthweight, affecting up to 5% of those under 1500 g. Candidaemia presents in a non-specific way; the infant shows the usual non-specific signs of sepsis. Fundoscopy is important since ocular candidiasis, both retinal and in the vitreous humour, has been reported in systemic candidiasis. Renal candidiasis may occur as part of a generalized candidaemia or as an isolated presentation with renal mass and partial or complete urinary obstruction. As bag specimens of urine are often contaminated from colonized skin, positive urines should be confirmed by suprapubic aspirate; renal ultrasound is valuable in identifying renal enlargement. Meningitis may occur; brain abscess is not usually recognized until autopsy. Osteomyelitis, septic arthritis and rarely cardiac vegetations have been described.

The single most important risk factor, other than low birthweight, for the development of systemic candidiasis is the duration of antibiotic therapy. Other risk factors are: the duration of parenteral nutrition, including fat emulsion; endotracheal intubation; umbilical and central venous catheterization; and surgical procedures. Catheter removal alone may clear candidaemia in up to 75% of cases (28), but systemic antifungal therapy is needed for meningitis and severe systemic infection. 5-Flucytosine (5-FC) should never be given alone, because of the rapid emergence of resistance. Amphotericin and 5-FC in combination are less toxic than is often thought, although care should be taken and 5-FC levels monitored. This combination is the treatment of choice in most cases (29).

Viruses

Noscomial virus infections have tended to receive relatively little attention in the paediatric literature, but may be responsible for considerable mortality and morbidity. Outbreaks of enterovirus infection are the exception and here the tendency has perhaps been to over-react (30). Echoviruses and coxsackieviruses may be acquired perinatally (vertical transmission), usually in the late summer and autumn. The mother may be ill with diarrhoea, rash, fever or sore throat at or near the time of delivery, and affected babies usually present at 3–5 days of age with non-specific signs of sepsis. Both can cause an aseptic meningitis, and echoviruses may cause a fulminant hepatitis with bleeding from disseminated intravascular coagulation, hepatomegaly and death from massive hepatic necrosis. The reported mortality from vertically acquired echovirus infections is over 60%, and is 83% for babies with severe hepatitis (31). Horizontal transmission can occur from a vertically infected baby or from staff or visitors with enterovirus infections. In most outbreaks the primary source of introduction into the nursery is by a baby with vertical infection, not an ill visitor or member of staff, but later transmission is usually by staff who subsequently become symptomatic. The attack rate for echovirus infections is 22–52% of susceptible babies in reported outbreaks (31), although as outbreaks are selectively reported the true rate may be considerably lower. Infants with nosocomial enterovirus infection usually have a much milder illness than those with vertical infection. Some develop meningitis, but most present with fever, rash, poor feeding, diarrhoea, apnoea or cough. Although there have been occasional reports of severe and even fatal horizontal infections (32), the mortality in all reported outbreaks until 1985 was only seven (3.4%) of 206 infected babies (31).

Coxsackieviruses have caused fewer neonatal problems than echoviruses in the UK and USA, but severe outbeaks of coxsackie B virus infections occurred in South African nurseries in the 1950s (33). Myocarditis was a frequent presentation, and there was a high mortality, with six babies dying in one outbreak (34). It was not clear from this report, however, how many of the babies had been vertically and how many horizontally infected. Kaplan et al. reported eight fatal cases of neonatal coxsackie B virus infection over an 11-year period and reviewed 33 culture-proven fatal cases in the literature (35), most of which were probably vertically acquired. They found myocarditis to be invariable, sometimes causing a fulminant death in heart failure, sometimes coming on secondarily after an initial mild illness. The risk of serious disease from nosocomial coxsackie B infection is uncertain, but almost certainly considerably lower than from vertical infection.

Perhaps because of the severe outbreak of echovirus 11 reported in Cambridge (32), there has been a tendency in the UK to recommend closure of neonatal wards and mass prophylaxis with human immunoglobulins, as soon as a diagnosis of enterovirus infection is made. Since babies with vertically transmitted infection are the usual index cases in outbreaks, early identification of such babies is essential, on the grounds of a peripartum maternal infection, often but not always in late summer or autumn, and the clinical presentation of a baby aged 3–5 days with sepsis or aseptic meningitis. The baby can then be isolated and vigorous hand-washing instituted, as well as the cohorting of staff who should not work if they develop an infection. Stools and throat swabs from mother and baby and CSF from the baby should be cultured for viruses; a typical enterovirus cytopathic effect is often visible within 2–3 days. We do not recommend widespread administration of immunoglobulins unless there is at least clinical evidence of spread of enterovirus infections and would not close a referral intensive care nursery without strong evidence of a severe outbreak, since this in itself may jeopardize babies to a greater extent than the virus (30).

Respiratory syncytial virus (RSV) has been described as causing nosocomial infections in the newborn (36). Classic bronchiolitis is rare and most babies present with apnoea, rhinitis, cough, fever or pulmonary infiltrates, while babies with chronic lung disease may require increased oxygen. The signs of nosocomial RSV infection are indistinguishable clinically from those due to other respiratory viruses, and simultaneous winter outbreaks of RSV and rhinovirus (37) and of RSV and parainfluenza virus type 3 infection (38) have been described, in which the babies could not be distinguished clinically. Influenza virus has been described as causing an outbreak with similar non-specific clinical features (39). Although it is often assumed that respiratory viruses are spread by inhalation of droplets, Hall and Douglas have shown that RSV can be transmitted on the hands of staff and inoculated via the nasal mucosa or conjunctiva by rubbing the nose or eyes (40). Staff members often develop colds and transmit viruses to babies. In the winter it is rarely possible to stop all staff with colds from working, so staff should pay attention to hand-washing after blowing or touching their noses. If staff have colds, they should wear masks, but even the use of masks, gowns and gloves does not always prevent staff becoming infected and transmitting infection to infants (40, 41).

Herpes simplex virus can cause devastating disease with a high mortality and morbidity. As for enterovirus infections and varicella, the babies most at risk are those born to mothers with active, primary (cervical) infection.

Table 3.6. *Late-onset pneumonia (after 48 h of age) (NICU, John Radcliffe Hospital, Oxford; 1.5.84–30.9.87)*

Organism*	Number of isolates†
Staphylococcus epidermidis	4 (0)
Pseudomonas spp.	3 (2)
Coliform	1 (1)
Streptococcus faecalis	1 (1)

Definite pneumonia: seven episodes.
*Isolated from endotracheal tube and blood cultures.
†Multiple isolates in parentheses.

NICU, neonatal intensive care unit.

Table 3.7. *Late-onset pneumonia (after 48 h of age) (NICU, John Radcliffe Hospital, Oxford; 1.5.84–30.9.87)*

Organism*		Number of isolates†
Gram-negative bacilli		30
Coliform	15	
Pseudomonas spp.	12	
Escherichia coli	2	
Acinetobacter spp.	1	
Staphylococcus aureus		5
Staphylococcus epidermidis		2
Group B streptococcus		1
Haemophilus influenzae		1
No organism		4
Total isolates		39

*Isolated from endotracheal tube cultures.
†Multiple isolates common.

NICU, neonatal intensive care unit.

The risk of nosocomial infection with HSV is very low, but the literature is unsatisfactory as to exactly what is the risk. Light reviewed reports from 1951 until 1977 and found only 24 cases of nosocomial infection, despite countless exposures (42). Thirteen babies apparently acquired infection from a mother with oral herpes or serological evidence of infection, and seven died. Some or all of these cases may have been perinatally rather than postnatally acquired, as high vaginal swabs were not cultured for viruses. Nine babies were thought to have acquired the infection from adults or older children, mostly hospital staff but once from a grandmother and once from the baby's sister; seven died. Two babies were cross-infected from other babies and in one of these cases, but in none of the others, DNA fingerprinting was performed and showed the viruses to be identical. It is difficult on the basis of this information to decide what should be done about mothers or staff with cold sores. Some authorities have recommended that mothers should be separated from their babies and staff should be off work until lesions have healed, but this has great implications for mother–baby relationships and staffing on very little evidence. Our recommendation is for mothers and staff with cold sores to be treated with topical 35% idoxuridine in dimethyl sulphoxide cream five times a day for a maximum of 3 days. Staff are not allowed to handle babies until they have been treated for 24 h. Mothers are not separated from their babies, but wear a mask for 24 h. Babies whose mothers have primary or recurrent HSV are isolated from other babies until the babies' viral culture results are available. Hand-washing is emphasized. This uneasy compromise is made in recognition of the paucity of information and the potential severity of infection.

Antibiotic treatment of suspected nosocomial infection

Treatment of potentially septic babies will depend to an extent on the nature of the presentation. Since in most units the duration, route of administration and type of antibiotic therapy will be different if the baby has meningitis, and because of the non-specific presentation of viral, bacterial and fungal meningitis, we recommend performing a lumbar puncture before starting antibiotics. Skin or wound infections are likely to be due to *Staph. aureus* but abscesses can also be caused by *Staph. epidermidis*, gram-negative organisms and fungi, and pus should always be obtained for microscopy and culture whenever possible.

Nosocomial pneumonia is often difficult to diagnose radiographically in artificially ventilated babies, since the appearance is mimicked by pulmonary oedema and haemorrhage. Endotracheal aspirate cultures provide somewhat dubious evidence of the organisms likely to be causing pneumonia, but blood cultures are rarely positive in pneumonia. Over a 40-month period in Oxford only seven episodes of late-onset (nosocomial) pneumonia were associated with bacteraemia (Table 3.6), and in 34 episodes blood cultures were sterile, the likely pathogenic organisms, often multiple, grown from the endotracheal tube being shown in Table 3.7. Although gram-negative bacilli predominated, staphylococci, both *Staph. aureus* and *Staph. epidermidis*, were also important. The treatment of pneumonia may be based on regular surveillance of endotracheal tube cultures or on a general antibiotic policy, such as that used for all sepsis, and there is growing evidence that endotracheal tube cultures are poorly predictive of the organisms causing sepsis. We have argued previously that it is rational to use an antibiotic policy for treatment of potential sepsis and that this policy should be based not so much on the nature and antibiotic sensitivity of organisms colonizing babies but on the organisms causing systemic sepsis and the outcome of those episodes (4, 13, 43). When the sickest babies are all colonized with, say, gentamicin-resistant gram-negative bacilli and there are cases of systemic sepsis occurring with these organisms, then if gentamicin had been used as the standard aminoglycoside for treating sepsis, it seems logical to change to another aminoglycoside at least for a period. It has been shown that, when the antibiotic pressure is removed, the resistant organisms gradually disappear and the preferred antibiotic may later be reinstated (44).

There is growing evidence that the old concept of a *course* of antibiotics is highly artificial and often inappropriate. In neonatal units, where, of necessity, there is a very low threshold for starting antibiotics, these can safely be stopped after 2–3 days if cultures are negative (45). Infected shunts should always be removed and infected central venous catheters usually, although if venous access is a problem and the baby is responding to antibiotics by the time cultures are positive, central venous catheters can sometimes be preserved.

Surveillance

There has been a vogue for extensive surveillance of the organisms colonizing babies in nurseries, but the organisms causing sepsis may correlate rather poorly with overall colonization patterns (12, 13). Furthermore, surveillance of colonization is expensive and time-consuming. I believe that, except for research purposes, widespread surveillance of colonization is largely unnecessary. It is far more important to be aware of the organisms causing systemic sepsis, so that antibiotic policies may be changed rapidly when necessary.

Prevention of nosocomial infections

Environment

Ideally there should be about 7.5–9 m^2 (80–100 sq. ft) of floor space between each intensive care cot, 4.5 m^2 (50 sq. ft) between intermediate care cots and 2 m^2 (20–25 sq. ft) between cots of term infants (5). There should be no more than eight to ten steps from any cot to a sink, and sinks should be designed not to spray and with taps operated by foot or knee.

Routine ward cleaning is with disinfectant detergents and vacated cots should be cleaned with an iodophor or quaternary disinfectant. Stethoscopes and laryngoscopes should be cleaned with an alcohol- or iodine-based disinfectant. Closed incubators need regular cleaning, and if they contain water for humidification, this should be changed frequently. Any equipment using water is particularly liable to contamination. Ventilator tubing, humidifiers and suction equipment require regular autoclaving and if nebulized therapy is given, the equipment should be autoclaved every 8–12 h.

Babies

The umbilical cord is a potential site of entry of infection and the decline in severe staphylococcal infections may at least in part be due to improved cord care. Bactericidal dyes such as triple dye and ointments containing bacitracin or sulphadiazine are more effective at suppressing bacteria but may keep the cord moist, and some prefer to use alcohol.

There has been some concern about possible neurotoxicity from bathing babies in hexachlorophene, and soap and sterile water are now preferred. Prophylaxis against gonococcal ophthalmia with topical silver nitrate, topical antibiotics (erythromycin or tetracycline) or even intramuscular penicillin G is advocated in the USA, but not practised in the UK.

Staff

Staffing levels are dictated by finances and politics, but it is clear that the incidence of nosocomial infections increases as staffing levels fall. Hand-washing is the most important infection-control measure. Soap and water for 15 seconds removes most superficial bacteria, while chlorhexidine or iodine-based soaps increase the effectiveness (46).

Masks and gloves are generally only needed for surgical procedures, although we recommend staff with colds should wear masks. Gowns are worn to feed babies and sterile gowns used for surgery. The situation when staff develop herpetic cold sores has been discussed and other illnesses should be considered on merit.

Mother

Nosocomial, as opposed to vertical, transmission from the mother is relatively uncommon. Similar considerations to those discussed for staff apply.

Visitors

Visiting has fortunately become increasingly open in intensive care nurseries and for psychological reasons it is preferable to allow free access to parents, siblings and grandparents and limited access to other relatives and friends. Visitors should wash their hands to the elbows before touching the baby and should not handle other babies without washing hands in between. All visitors, especially children, with respiratory infections should be asked not to visit until they have recovered. Despite wider visiting, nosocomial virus infections are relatively uncommon, even in winter months (47).

Isolation

It has often been customary to isolate babies with diseases such as bacterial meningitis, septicaemia, pneumonia or urinary-tract infection who are in fact at low risk of transmitting infection to other babies. Infants who should be isolated are those with diarrhoea, with suspected enterovirus infection and with congenital rubella. Syphilis, gonococcal and possibly chlamydial conjunctivitis are also possible contagious conditions. *L. monocytogenes* has occasionally caused serious nosocomial infection and babies and their mothers should probably be isolated, whereas group B streptococci have rarely caused infection and isolation is unnecessary.

Isolation of affected babies is important in outbreaks of diarrhoea, whether due to bacteria or viruses, and in outbreaks of enterovirus infection.

Cohorting

Cohorting of babies and staff may be used to limit spread of infection. Babies born over a given period, say 24 h, are nursed together in one part of the nursery and by the same staff, limiting spread among babies, especially that transmitted by staff. This can be useful when there is a heavy workload and when there is a potentially serious organism circulating in the nursery.

Prophylactic antibiotics

There is a very limited role for prophylactic antibiotics in the neonatal unit. They have not been shown to reduce infection due to umbilical catheters, central venous catheters or endotracheal intubation. In adults undergoing bowel surgery there is evidence that antibiotics effective against gram-positive and gram-negative organisms, such as cefuroxime, given at anaesthetic induction, reduce the incidence of postoperative sepsis. They have been used for neonates, although without formal proof of their efficacy. Antistaphylococcal antibiotics at the time of insertion of ventricular shunts are often used, but are of unproven efficacy.

Immunotherapy

The use of intramuscular or IV immunoglobulins prophylactically to reduce nosocomial infections is unproven, but under investigation.

Miscellaneous

Early enteral feeding of babies, by reducing the need for indwelling cannulas, will lead to a decrease in sepsis, particularly due to staphylococci. A strict antibiotic policy with regular review of the need for antibiotics in each baby can reduce the amount of antibiotics used and reduce the selection pressure for resistant bacteria. Constant reminders on ward rounds about hand-washing between handling babies and after scratching noses or beards, and a greater understanding about the factors involved in nosocomial infection, can all help to reduce infection in a unit.

Summary

Nosocomial infections have a lower mortality than vertically transmitted bacterial and viral infections, but cause significant morbidity, often prolonging hospital stay. To a certain extent, given the extreme vulnerability of the population at risk in terms of immunological immaturity and life-saving but invasive interventions, nosocomial infections are inevitable. Nevertheless, they can be kept to a minimum by good infection-control practice and so are, at least to an extent, preventable.

References

1. Hoogkamp-Korstanje JAA, Cats B, Senders RC, van Ertbruggen I. Analysis of bacterial infections in a neonatal intensive care unit. J Hosp Infection 1982; 3: 275–84.
2. Goldmann DA, Durbin WA, Freeman J. Nosocomial infections in a neonatal intensive care unit. J Infect Dis 1981; 144: 449–59.
3. Haley RW, Bregman DA. The role of understaffing and overcrowding in recurrent outbreaks of staphylococcal infection in a neonatal special-care baby unit. J Infect Dis 1982; 45: 875–85.

4. Isaacs D, Catterson J, Hope PL, Moxon ER, Wilkinson AR. Factors influencing colonisation with gentamicin-resistant gram negative organisms in the neonatal unit. Arch Dis Child 1988; 63: 533–5.
5. Nelson JD. Control of infection acquired in the nursery. In: Remington JS, Klein JO (eds). Infectious diseases of the fetus and newborn infant. 2nd ed. Philadelphia: WB Saunders, 1983: 1035–52.
6. Balagtas RC, Bell CE, Edwards LD, Levin S. Risk of local and systemic infections associated with umbilical vein catheterization: a prospective study in 86 newborn patients. Pediatrics 1971; 48: 359–67.
7. Bard H, Albert G, Teasdale F, Doray B, Martineau B. Prophylactic antibiotics in chronic umbilical artery catheterisation. Arch Dis Child 1973; 48: 630–5.
8. van Vliet PJ, Gupta JM. Prophylactic antibiotics in umbilical artery catheterisation in the newborn. Arch Dis Child 1973; 48: 296–300.
9. Parvey LS, Ch'ien LT. Neonatal herpes simplex virus infection introduced by fetal monitor scalp electrodes. Pediatrics 1980; 96: 824–8.
10. Goldmann DA, Leclair J, Macone A. Bacterial colonization of neonates admitted to an intensive care environment. J Pediatr 1978; 93: 288–93.
11. McGowan JE Jr, Barnes MW, Finland M. Bacteremia at Boston City Hospital: occurrence and mortality during 12 selected years (1935–1972), with special reference to hospital-acquired cases. J Infect Dis 1975; 132: 316–35.
12. White RED, Townsend TR, Stephens MA, Moxon ER. Are surveillance of resistant enteric bacilli and antimicrobial usage among neonates in a newborn intensive care unit useful? Pediatrics 1981; 68: 1–4.
13. Isaacs D, Wilkinson AR, Moxon ER. Surveillance of colonisation and late-onset septicaemia in neonates. J Hosp Infect 1987; 10: 114–19.
14. Adams BG, Marrie TJ. Hand carriage of aerobic gram-negative rods may not be transient. J Hyg 1982; 89: 33–46.
15. Challacombe D. Bacterial microflora in infants receiving nasojejunal tube feeding. J Pediatr 1974; 85: 113 (letter).
16. Morrison AJ, Wenzel RP. Epidemiology of infections due to *Pseudomonas aeruginosa*. Rev Infect Dis 1984; 6: S627–42.
17. Brumfitt W, Dixson S, Hamilton-Miller JMT. Resistance to antiseptics in methicillin and gentamicin resistant *Staphylococcus aureus*. Lancet 1985; 1: 422–3.
18. Hall RT, Hall SL, Barnes WG, Izuegbu J, Rogolsky M, Zorbas I. Characteristics of coagulase-negative staphylococci from infants with bacteremia. Pediatr Infect Dis J 1987; 6: 377–83.
19. Hensey OJ, Hart CA, Cooke RWI. Serious infection in a neonatal intensive care unit: a two-year survey. J Hyg 1985; 95: 289–97.
20. Fleer A, Senders RC, Visser MR et al. Septicemia due to coagulase negative staphylococci in a neonatal intensive care unit: clinical and bacteriological features and contaminated parenteral fluids as a source of sepsis. Pediatr Infect Dis J 1983; 2: 426–31.
21. Kirpalani H, Schmidt B, Ford-Jones L, Corey M, Philip AGS. Are coagulase negative staphylococci (CNS) true pathogens in newborn infants? A concurrent cohort study. Paper presented at the Annual Meeting of the British Paediatric Association, York, 1986.
22. Anthony BF, Okada DM, Hobel CJ. Epidemiology of the group B streptococcus: maternal and nosocomial sources for infant acquisitions. J Pediatr 1979; 95: 431–6.
23. Paredes A, Wong P, Mason EO, Taber LH, Barrett FF. Nosocomial transmission of group B streptococci in a nursery. Pediatrics 1977; 59: 679–82.
24. Steere AC, Aber RC, Warford LR et al. Possible nosocomial transmission of group B streptococci in a newborn nursery. J Pediatr 1975; 87: 784–7.
25. Pass MA, Gray BM, Khare S, Dillon HC. Prospective studies of group B streptococcal infections in infants. J Pediatr 1979; 95: 437–43.
26. Dennis JE, Rhodes KH, Cooney DR, Roberts GD. Nosocomial *Rhizopus* infection (zygomycosis) in children. J Pediatr 1980; 96: 824–8.
27. Murphy N, Buchanan CR, Damjanovic V, Whitaker R, Hart CA, Cooke RWI. Infection and colonisation of neonates by *Hansenula anomala*. Lancet 1986; 1: 291–3.
28. Weese-Mayer DE, Fondriest DW, Brouillette RT, Shulman ST. Risk factors associated with candidemia in the neonatal intensive care unit: a case-control study. Pediatr Infect Dis J 1987; 6: 190–6.
29. Baley J, Klegman R, Fanaroff A. Disseminated fungal infections in very low birthweight infants: clinical manifestations and epidemiology. Pediatrics 1984; 73: 144–52.

30. Isaacs D, Dobson SRM, Wilkinson AR, Hope PL, Eglin R, Moxon ER. Conservative management of an echovirus 11 outbreak in a neonatal unit. Lancet 1989; 1: 543–5.
31. Modlin JF. Perinatal echovirus infection: insights from a literature review of 61 cases of serious infection and 16 outbreaks in nurseries. Rev Infect Dis 1986; 8: 918–26.
32. Nagington J, Wreghitt TG, Gandy G, Roberton NRC, Berry PJ. Fatal echovirus 11 infections in outbreak in special care baby unit. Lancet 1978; 2: 725–8.
33. Editorial. Avoiding the danger of enteroviruses to newborn infants. Lancet 1986; 1: 194–5.
34. Javett SN, Heymann S, Mundel B et al. Myocarditis in the newborn infant: a study of an outbreak associated with coxsackie group B virus infection in a maternity home in Johannesburg. Pediatrics 1956; 48: 1–22.
35. Kaplan MH, Klein SW, McPhee J, Harper RG. Group B coxsackievirus infections in infants younger than three months of age: a serious childhood illness. Rev Infect Dis 1983; 5: 1019–32.
36. Hall CB, Kopelman AE, Douglas RG Jr, Geiman JM, Meagher MP. Neonatal respiratory syncytial virus infection. N Engl J Med 1979; 300: 393–6.
37. Valent WM, Clarke TA, Hall CB, Memegus MA, Shapiro DL. Concurrent outbreaks of rhinovirus and respiratory syncytial virus in an intensive care nursery. J Pediatr 1982; 100: 722–6.
38. Meissner HC, Murray SA, Kiernan MA, Snydaman DR, McIntosh K. A simultaneous outbreak of respiratory syncytial virus and parainfluenza virus type 3 in a newborn nursery. J Pediatr 1984; 104: 680–4.
39. Meibalane R, Sedmak GV, Sasidharan P, Garg P, Grausz JP. Outbreak of influenza in a neonatal intensive care unit. J Pediatr 1977; 91: 974–6.
40. Hall CB, Douglas RG. Modes of transmission of respiratory syncytial virus. J Pediatr 1981; 99: 100–3.
41. Murphy D, Todd JK, Chao RK, Orr I, McIntosh K. The use of gowns and masks to control respiratory illness in pediatric hospital personnel. J Pediatr 1981; 99: 746–50.
42. Light IJ. Postnatal acquisition of herpes simplex virus by the newborn infant: a review of the literature. Pediatrics 1979; 63: 480–2.
43. Isaacs D, Wilkinson AR. Antibiotic use in the neonatal unit. Arch Dis Child 1987; 62: 204–8.
44. Franco JA, Eitzman DV, Baer H. Antibiotic usage and microbial resistance in an intensive care nursery. Am J Dis Child 1973; 126: 318–21.
45. Isaacs D, Wilkinson AR, Moxon ER. Duration of antibiotic courses of neonates. Arch Dis Child 1987; 62: 727–8.
46. Sprunt K, Redman W, Leidy F. Antibacterial effectiveness of routine hand-washing. Pediatrics 1973; 52: 264–7.
47. Rudd PT, Carrington D. A prospective study of chlamydial, mycoplasmal and viral infections in a neonatal intensive care unit. Arch Dis Child 1984; 59: 120–5.

4 Diagnostic Tests for Bacterial Infection in the Newborn

A. G. S. Philip
Division of Neonatology,
Maine Medical Center, Portland and
University of Vermont College of Medicine, USA

Abstract

Proof of bacterial infection is provided by positive cultures; however, this may take 24–48 h, and so multiple tests have been used in attempts to reach an earlier diagnosis. No single test has emerged as being completely reliable. The test with the greatest sensitivity seems to be the immature to total neutrophil quotient (I/T). More than 90% of infected neonates have an increased I/T at initial investigation. Unfortunately, other circumstances (such as asphyxia) may also increase I/T, and therefore the test lacks specificity. Other tests have high positive predictive value (when the test is positive, infection is likely) and the best of these seems to be C-reactive protein (CRP). When CRP exceeds 20 mg/l, infection is very probable.

These tests may also be used to guide antibiotic therapy. With negative cultures and no test values abnormal by 48 h after culture, antibiotics may be stopped with confidence. The perfect test remains elusive, but the search continues.

Introduction

Bacterial infection in the newborn may be superficial and localized (such as conjunctivitis, omphalitis and pustules), deep and localized, or systemic (such as septicaemia, meningitis, pneumonia, septic arthritis and osteomyelitis). Diagnosis of superficial infections is usually easy, but generalized infections present a major diagnostic challenge because of the multiplicity of risk factors and clinical manifestations (1). The only certain way of diagnosing bacterial sepsis and meningitis is to have positive cultures, but this is where we encounter the primary problem.

> *Primary problem*
> Culture diagnosis takes 24–28 h, *but* delay in antibiotic administration may result in increased mortality and morbidity.

In addition there are certain situations which mitigate against obtaining positive cultures. This is a secondary problem.

> *Secondary problem*
> Positive cultures may not be obtained, because *either* the mother received antibiotics before delivery *or* the baby was treated before referral.

Thus there is a need for diagnostic tests which will allow a presumptive diagnosis of systemic infection to be made.

Infection in the Newborn. Edited by J. de Louvois and D. Harvey
©1990 John Wiley & Sons Ltd

> . . . the clinician who later uses the test starts with patients whose condition is unknown. The purpose of the test is to predict (or identify) what the patient's condition really is. In receiving the result of the test, an investigator therefore wants to know its predictive accuracy, not its sensitivity or specificity . . .
>
> . . . the predictive value will depend entirely on the ratio of confirmed positive and confirmed negative people to whom the test was applied . . .
>
> . . . if patients are chosen merely because they do or do not have the target disease, the discrimination of the test will not be adequately evaluated . . . to deal with clinical reality requires a confrontation with clinical complexity . . .
>
> Feinstein (2)

Although a large number of diagnostic tests have been evaluated, no single test has sufficiently high sensitivity and specificity to allow it to be relied upon. From a clinical point of view, positive predictive value (how likely infection is, with a positive test) is the more useful way of approaching a test. Even a combination of tests has not yielded 100% sensitivity or positive predictive value, so the search for the ideal test or tests continues. This is particularly true for early-onset infection, especially within 12 h of birth. This review will deal with currently available tests and will describe those that are most valuable.

Diagnostic tests which appear to be valuable

It has been suggested that high sensitivity is needed if a disease is serious but treatable, and high positive predictive value is needed if treatment of a false positive might have serious consequences (3). Indiscriminate antibiotic use can lead to emergence of resistant organisms, with potentially lethal consequences. Thus tests with high sensitivity and positive predictive value have been sought.

Leucocyte counts

Increasing reliance has been placed in the last decade on the white blood cell count (WBC) and differential count, based on a number of studies performed in the 1970s. Useful standards for the neutrophil series were provided by Manroe et al. in 1979 (4). In addition, morphological abnormalities of the neutrophils were emphasized by Zipursky et al. (5).

Absolute leucocyte counts may be more useful than absolute neutrophil counts (1), although the normal range is wide (from $5.0–30.0 \times 10^9/l$ in the first week). This is of practical importance, since absolute leucocyte counts are reported by the laboratory, whereas neutrophil counts may require calculation from differential percentages. Absolute neutropenia (less than $1.0 \times 10^9/l$) is quite predictive of bacterial infection, but not very sensitive. Both leucocyte counts and neutrophil counts normally increase during the first 12 h after birth and decline again by 24–36 h after birth (4). When direction of change is markedly opposite to what would be expected, bacterial infection should be strongly suspected (6).

Interpretation of most leucocyte counts requires caution. Several factors have been noted to affect the results significantly. For instance, asphyxia and maternal hypertension may increase the absolute numbers of total neutrophils and immature neutrophils (4). The method of blood sampling influences the counts, as do birthweight and gestational age (1).

By far the most sensitive test for detecting most bacterial infections is the immature to total neutrophil quotient or ratio (I/T). However, despite its sensitivity (likelihood of a positive test with documented infection), it is not particularly predictive. This has been exaggerated by a change in the standards for reporting 'bands' (the most usual immature neutrophils to be seen). It was previously shown that the upper limit of I/T was 0.17, and values equal to or greater than 0.2 have been used to designate a 'positive' test. With a more liberal interpretation of what constitutes a 'band' (or 'stab') form, a positive test should probably be equal to or greater than 0.3. The I/T quotient seems to be less affected by birthweight and gestational age, but can still be increased by asphyxia and other haematological stress. It may also be within normal limits in cases of sepsis associated with coagulase-negative staphylococci (7) and even in occasional cases of group B streptococcal infection (8). Most reports of the value of I/T have dealt with early-onset infection. It may be that lower quotients can be used in neonates older than 1 week of age.

There is comparatively little information about morphological abnormalities of white blood cells, but the presence of toxic granulation, vacuolated polymorphonuclear cells and Döhle bodies has been considered predictive of infection (5). Personal observations suggest that these findings are not a very sensitive indicator of infection, but have quite a high positive predictive value.

C-reactive protein

During the acute phase of the inflammatory response, several plasma proteins increase in concentration, while others may decrease (9). Among these *acute-phase proteins*, C-reactive protein (CRP) seems to be the most acutely responsive. Because in most normal infants and adults CRP levels are barely detectable, increased CRP levels are easily demonstrated. An additional advantage of using CRP as an index is that concentrations may increase to many times normal levels (up to 100 times or more).

The first studies to report the value of CRP in diagnosing neonatal infection used a rapid qualitative technique, where the test was reported as positive or negative. A positive test using latex-particle agglutination (LPA) was roughly equivalent to a plasma CRP concentration greater than 10 mg/l. Quantitative determinations were possible with radial immunodiffusion, but this takes 24 h or so. The study by Sabel and Hanson in 1974 (10) suggested that CRP might be quite valuable, and in 1979 Sabel and Wadsworth demonstrated that sensitivity could be as high as 89% for sepsis and meningitis (11). More recent studies suggest that such sensitivity is unlikely at the time of initial evaluation for sepsis, particularly when cases of very early-onset infection are evaluated, especially with group B streptococcal infection (12).

It is now possible to perform rapid quantitative determinations using a variety of techniques (9). While quantitation is desirable in hospitals equipped to measure CRP quantitatively, it is possible to obtain a close approximation by using serial dilutions with the LPA method (13). Such determinations provide semi-quantitative values which could be obtained in any hospital. There appears to be some correlation between the maximum level of CRP and the severity of illness, but there also seems to be some variability of response with different bacteria; for example, a marked increase in CRP usually accompanies infection with *Escherichia coli*, whereas some infants with sepsis due to coagulase-negative staphylococci have a very limited CRP response (7). Further information on this would be valuable.

Acute-phase proteins (APPs) increase with inflammation or tissue necrosis. Since the most usual reason for inflammation in the neonate is bacterial infection, CRP has proved valuable in diagnosing systemic infection. However, it should be remembered that there are other reasons for an increase in CRP in the neonatal period. These include meconium-aspiration syndrome (14) (presumably secondary to chemical pneumonitis), proven cases of necrotizing enterocolitis (15, 16) and the inflammatory response of the early postoperative period (first 3 or 4 days) in infants undergoing surgical procedures. On the other hand, personal observations indicate minimal or no increase in infants with chest tubes, no increase with umbilical artery catheters and no increase with periventricular–intraventricular haemorrhage.

Some authors indicate that levels of CRP may be between 10 and 20 mg/l in the first day or so after birth (17). Whether this is in some way related to inflammation of the umbilical stump is uncertain. What seems clear is that, when CRP is greater than 20 mg/l, almost all neonates will have demonstrable infection (personal observations) if there is no evidence of meconium aspiration. In the few who have a raised CRP in the absence of positive cultures, pneumonia and osteomyelitis, there is experimental evidence to support the idea that the CRP elevation could be caused by circulating endotoxin (18). There is also clinical evidence of a sepsis-like picture caused by endotoxin without demonstrable bacteraemia (19), and limited clinical information documenting increased levels of CRP with endotoxinaemia and sepsis (20).

Erythrocyte sedimentation rate

Until recently, the most widely used indicator of acute infection was the erythrocyte sedimentation rate (ESR). Erythrocyte sedimentation is primarily determined by the level of fibrinogen, although haematocrit is also a factor. Increased levels of fibrinogen (and decreased haematocrit) produce increased ESR. The traditional methods of measuring ESR (Westergren and Wintrobe) use larger amounts of blood than are reasonable in small neonates. Consequently, techniques using smaller samples of blood have been devised, the most popular being the mini-ESR (mESR), which uses a micro-haematocrit tube (21).

In contrast to CRP, which seems to increase within 8–12 h of the onset of infection, mESR is frequently within normal limits for 24 h or more (1). Nevertheless, mESR levels equal to or greater than 10 mm/h in the first 24 h, or more than 15 mm/h after this time, are strongly suggestive of infection when the haematocrit is over 40%. In other words, sensitivity is poor, but positive predictive value is high.

As with all acute-phase proteins, other causes of inflammation will produce an increase in ESR. In addition, haemolytic disease of the newborn due to ABO incompatibility has been associated with increased ESR. In contrast, decreased ESR is observed in cases of infection associated with disseminated intravascular coagulation, because of decreased fibrinogen levels.

Other APPs

A number of other proteins have been evaluated in neonatal infection, but almost all have limitations similar to those of the ESR. The most useful of these other APPs seems to be alpha-1-acid glycoprotein (AGP) (orosomucoid) (22, 23). Because the upper limit of normal seems to vary with gestation and age after delivery, interpretation is more difficult than with CRP. Some authors have reported AGP to be valuable in early diagnosis of neonatal sepsis, but it seems to be more useful in documenting persistence of inflammation. Thus it may be helpful in deciding when to discontinue antibiotics.

Other APPs reported to be valuable are fibrinogen, haptoglobin and alpha-1-antitrypsin; they increase in some circumstances, but accumulated experience suggests that they are not particularly sensitive or predictive (1). Proteins which decrease with neonatal infection are pre-albumin, transferrin and fibronectin. However, this decrease is not sufficiently consistent to allow use in early diagnosis.

Other non-specific tests

Several other tests initially seemed promising, but have not provided consistent results. Immunoglobulin M seems to increase only after about 48 h; platelets are rarely decreased in the first 24 h; the nitroblue tetrazolium test is variable and dependent upon adequate numbers of neutrophils; and the buffy-coat examination for engulfed bacteria is also affected by neutropenia and can be quite tedious to perform.

Combination of tests

With the realization that single tests had their limitations, I formulated the idea (a little over a decade ago) that a combination of simple, rapid and cheap tests might provide the most valuable approach. In 1980, I described a system that used five tests in combination (24). Positive tests were:

(1) WBC $< 5.0 \times 10^9$/l
(2) I/T $\geqslant 0.2$
(3) mESR $\geqslant 15$ mm/h
(4) latex CRP positive
(5) latex haptoglobin positive.

If two or more tests were positive, infection was very likely. I called this a *sepsis screen*. In an update in 1982 (25), for 524 infants tested in the first week, the sepsis screen had a positive predictive value for septicaemia of 39% and for infection (septicaemia, pneumonia, etc.) of 68%. This should be compared to an incidence of 8% for septicaemia and 14% for infection. In other words, the ability to predict infection was improved about five times (compared to guessing). Between 8 and 60 days ($n = 56$), the sepsis screen had a positive predictive value of 46% for septicaemia and 78% for infection (25).

A modification of this sepsis screen was recently described, substituting fibronectin testing for haptoglobin (26). The addition of the fibronectin test did not improve the positive predictive value compared to using the other four tests together. Recent personal experience suggests that a combination of total WBC, I/T and quantitative CRP may be sufficient in the vast majority of cases. Similar findings have been noted using only I/T and quantitative CRP in another recent report which prospectively evaluated 250 consecutive neonatal admissions to a regional perinatal referral centre (27). This report and our own experience suggest that CRP levels may frequently not be increased at initial evaluation, whereas I/T is almost always positive.

These results with combinations of tests are quite encouraging and might be further enhanced by additional consideration of specific clinical features. Further evaluation of this approach is needed from different centres and should take different ages at evaluation into account.

Detection of bacterial antigen

In addition to the non-specific tests noted previously, certain specific bacteria may be detected by using countercurrent immunoelectrophoresis (CIE) or latex particle agglutination (LPA). The detection of bacterial antigen is easier with LPA, and urine seems to be the most reliable body fluid for this purpose. Unfortunately, there may be a considerable delay in obtaining urine from sick babies, but LPA has been particularly valuable for detecting group B streptococcal antigen (28, 29). There is also a commercial reagent for *E. coli* K_1 antigen, but little information has been published on its value. Other available test-kits are not usually applicable to the newborn.

Recently evaluated tests

There are a number of other non-specific tests which have been evaluated recently and which may prove to be useful; however, these will require further study to determine whether they are superior to the simple tests now employed.

Elastase-alpha-1-proteinase inhibitor

Early experience suggests that this test is the most likely to displace current tests. Levels in infected neonates appear to be clearly above those in controls and do not seem to be affected by leucopenia or neutropenia (30, 31). These increased levels may appear before an increase in CRP.

Alpha-amylase

This test has been described recently in healthy and infected neonates. The mean value for the infected group was markedly decreased compared to the mean value for the healthy group. However, there was considerable overlap between the two groups (32).

Chemiluminescence

This is another test which involves the white blood cells. This test estimates granulocyte phagocytic activity, which is depressed to a variable extent by different organisms (33). It can be measured within 15 min. Further experience is required in other populations.

Complement

The main metabolite of the third component of complement is C3d. Using a qualitative test, the positive predictive value of C3d was 44% for infection among 19 babies with infection and 110 without evidence of infection (34). Further studies, possibly using this test in combination with others, seem warranted.

Management

The clinical picture of neonatal sepsis may be so overwhelming that there is no doubt in the clinician's mind about the diagnosis. However, occasional babies fool us into thinking they are infected when they have metabolic diseases or other life-threatening disorders. It seems reasonable to make the occasional mistake and to begin antibiotics under these circumstances.

However, in other situations there are two possible solutions to the problems posed earlier.

Solution A

Treat with antibiotics every baby with risk factors or clinical manifestations suggesting systemic infection: but for how long?

(a) until clinically well *or*
(b) 7, 10, 14 or 21 days (arbitrary lengths of time)?

Solution A may lead to:

(1) emergence of resistant organisms;
(2) increased costs;
(3) lack of thought about individual babies.

Solution B

Attempt to evaluate term infants before antibiotic treatment (especially those with 'risk' factors only). Evaluate preterm infants during first 48 h after cultures have been taken and antibiotic treatment started.

Solution B may occasionally lead to delay in treating an infected term infant.

I favour Solution B. Evaluation may be performed with the diagnostic tests noted earlier. If WBC and differential counts are within normal limits and there is no increase in CRP during the first 24–48 h, antibiotics may be discontinued at 48 h with confidence (provided cultures are negative).

If the mother is treated with antibiotics before delivery, or the baby is referred without obtaining blood for culture before starting antibiotics, evaluating urine for bacterial antigen may be helpful in addition to the other tests. In babies with an endotracheal tube in place, a positive culture

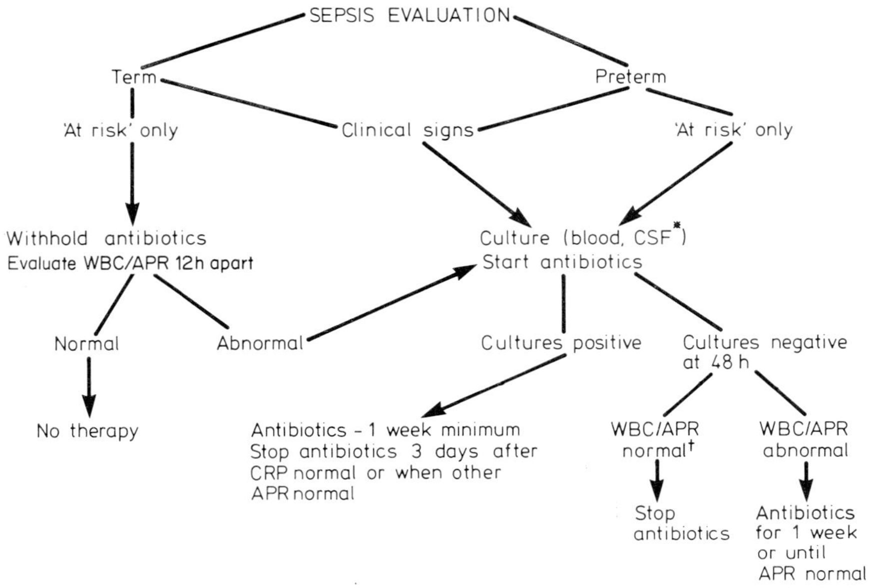

Fig. 4.1. Approach to antibiotic therapy. *and urine after 3 days. †Three values in first 48 h. APR, acute-phase reactants; CRP, C-reactive protein; WBC, white blood cells; CSF, cerebrospinal fluid.

Table 4.1. *Listeria pneumonia: mother treated before delivery*

Baby boy B. 1650 g/32 weeks. Preterm labour; maternal fever (38.6 °C) night before. Pus from cervix; ampicillin prior to delivery. Apgar 1/4; scattered petechiae, poor perfusion, hypotension (corrected).

Date	WBC ($\times 10^9$/l)	I/T ratio	Platelets ($\times 10^9$/l)	CRP (mg/l)
4.1.86	9.4	58/65 (0.89)	174	70
5.1.86	12.8	59/77 (0.77)	Mod. decrease	101
6.1.86	25.5	21/89 (0.24)	45	112
7.1.86	30.4	31/90 (0.34)	21; 45	66
8.1.86	36.5	21/86 (0.24)	69	42
9.1.86	41.5	24/82 (0.29)	55	24
10.1.86	48.9	22/80 (0.28)	152	9
12.1.86	61.6	39/77 (0.51)	—	<6
14.1.86	33.8	16/64 (0.25)	—	<6
17.1.86	22.2	10/78 (0.13)	—	<6

Gastric aspirate/tracheal aspirate: *Listeria monocytogenes*.

Intraventricular haemorrhage with dilated ventricles. Assisted ventilation for 7 days.

WBC, white blood cell count; I/T, immature/total neutrophils; CRP, C-reactive protein.

of endotracheal aspirate in conjunction with radiographic changes is strong presumptive evidence of pneumonia (35) and may be supported by leucocyte and CRP values.

Since CRP values decrease rapidly with appropriate antibiotic management, it may be wise to continue antibiotics for an additional 2 or 3 days after CRP is normal, or until other APPs (e.g. AGP) have returned to normal. It certainly seems unwise to stop antibiotics in the face of elevated levels of CRP in infants with meningitis (or other systemic infection) since relapse has been reported in these circumstances (10).

Another approach to the problem of early-onset infection is to develop tests in the mother which are highly predictive of infection in the baby. At present, the yield of proven neonatal infection from *risk* situations suggesting amniotic fluid infection is remarkably low (1). This approach is currently under investigation.

In the absence of strong clinical predictors of infection, it is necessary to evaluate infants born to mothers with possible amniotic fluid infection and infants with a wide variety of clinical manifestations. The tests described can help to diagnose infected babies, can

Table 4.2. *Klebsiella sepsis: older infant*

Baby boy P. Twin 'B'; 700 g/28 weeks. Age: 6 weeks. Abdominal distension; apnoea.

Date	WBC ($\times 10^9$/l)	I/T ratio	Platelets ($\times 10^9$/l)	CRP (mg/l)
17.9.85	3.6	45/53 (0.85)	Normal	119
18.9.85	7.6	24/44 (0.55)	126	151
19.9.85	7.8	10/54 (0.19)	Slight decrease	81
20.9.85	7.7	15/44 (0.34)	Slight decrease	41
22.9.85	11.9	11/51 (0.22)	—	12
24.9.85				<6

Blood culture: *Klebsiella pneumoniae.*

WBC, white blood cell count; I/T, immature/total neutrophils; CRP, C-reactive protein.

Table 4.3. *Pneumococcal pneumonia: preterm infant*

Baby boy S. 1780 g/32 weeks. Rupture of membranes 48 h; maternal temperature 38.1 °C; caesarian section (fetal distress). Apgar 1/7; hypotension.

Date	WBC ($\times 10^9$/l)	I/T ratio	CRP (mg/l)
20.11.85 a.m.	5.2	17/27 (0.63)	15
p.m.	6.9	55/67 (0.82)	
21.11.85	10.8	46/73 (0.63)	50
22.11.84	15.9	12/89 (0.13)	27
23.11.85			9
25.11.85			<6

Gastric aspirate/tracheal aspirate: *Streptococcus pneumoniae.*

Assisted ventilation for 5 days. Chest X-ray: Pneumonia.

WBC, white blood cell count; I/T, immature/total neutrophils; CRP, C-reactive protein.

Table 4.4. *Devastating pneumococcal sepsis and meningitis (late onset): term infant*

Baby girl J. 3 kg/term. Age: 11 days. 9.5.85: apnoea–meningitis diagnosed (other hospital). 11.5.85: seizures–transfer initiated.

Date	WBC ($\times 10^9$/l)	I/T ratio	CRP (mg/l)	EEG
9.5.85*	27.1	25/70 (0.36)		
11.5.85	29.7	23/57 (0.40)	168	
12.5.85	26.5	27/75 (0.36)	134	
13.5.85				Burst suppression
15.5.85				Flat
24.5.85	17.2	19/44 (0.43)	52	
2.6.85	18.3	14/27 (0.52)	56	

*Data from other hospital.

Blood and cerebrospinal fluid: *Streptococcus pneumoniae.*

Assisted ventilation for 7 days. Severe encephalomalacia with liquefaction (seen on ultrasound).

WBC, white blood cell count; I/T, immature/total neutrophils; CRP, C-reactive protein; EEG, electroencephalogram.

Table 4.5. *Group B streptococcus (GBS) sepsis: term infant.*

Baby Boy D. Born 30.10.87. 3150 g/38 weeks. Rupture of membranes 26 h. Apgar 8/9. Three hours postdelivery: grunting, tachypnoea, pallor, cyanosis. Chest X-ray: widespread infiltrate; right pleural effusion. Required 40% oxygen.

Date	WBC ($\times 10^9$/l)	I/T ratio	CRP (mg/l)	
30.10.87	26.0	12/58 (0.21)	21	Bacterial antigen: GBS
31.10.87	31.0	18/80 (0.23)	35	Blood culture: GBS
1.11.87	34.8	11/67 (0.16)	27	Gastric aspirate: GBS
2.11.87			13	
3.11.87			12	
9.11.87			<10	Antibiotics: 10 days

WBC, white blood cell count; I/T, immature/total neutrophils; CRP, C-reactive protein.

Table 4.6. *Group B streptococcus (GBS) infection: mother treated before delivery*

Baby boy E. Born 8.11.87. 3720 g/40 weeks. Rupture of membranes 7 h; maternal fever (39.5 °C), chills/shivering. Fetal tachycardia (200/min); meconium-stained amniotic fluid. Ampicillin to mother before delivery (caesarian section). Apgar $3^1/5^5/8^{10}$; endotracheal tube suction $\times$ 4. Initially, baby required 60% oxygen, but improved rapidly.

Date		WBC ($\times 10^9$/l)	I/T ratio	CRP (mg/l)	
8.11.87	5 a.m.	9.1	30/59 (0.51)	<10	Gastric aspirate: GBS
	3 p.m.	13.5	29/57 (0.51)	30	Blood culture: no growth
9.11.87	8 a.m.	15.3	27/70 (0.39)	51	Bacterial antigen: GBS
10.11.87		10.8	14/59 (0.24)		
11.11.87		10.3	8/35 (0.23)	14	

WBC, white blood cell count; I/T, immature/total neutrophils; CRP, C-reactive protein.

Table 4.7. *Group B streptococcus (GBS) colonization: baby evaluated; antibiotics withheld*

Baby boy D. Born 14.10.86. Cystitis; rupture of membranes 9.10.86; GBS cultured from cervix. Gestation 38 weeks; maternal CRP <10 mg/l on 11.10.86 and 12.10.86, 11 mg/l on 13.10.86 and 14 mg/l on 14.10.86. Caesarian section (breech); birthweight = 3.02 kg; Apgar 9/9.

Date	WBC ($\times 10^9$/l)	I/T ratio	CRP (mg/l)
14.10.86	16.7	10/48 (0.21)	<10
15.10.86	15.3	9/53 (0.17)	<10
16.10.86	12.0	10/41 (0.24)	<10

Gastric: 1 + polymorphs on smear; cultures: blood and cerebrospinal fluid — no growth at 48 h.

WBC, white blood cell count; I/T, immature/total neutrophils; CRP, C-reactive protein.

certainly help to limit the duration of antibiotic administration in non-infected babies and may help in deciding how long antibiotics should be administered to infected neonates. This scheme is illustrated diagrammatically in Fig. 4.1.

Clinical examples

To illustrate the fact that this scheme can be used in clinical practice, I have provided examples of several cases of infected neonates seen at the Maine Medical Center in the last year or two (Tables 4.1–4.7).

References

1. Philip AGS. Neonatal sepsis and meningitis, Boston: GK Hall, 1985.
2. Feinstein AR. Clinical biostatistics XXXI: on the sensitivity, specificity and discrimination of diagnostic tests. Clin Pharmacol Ther 1975; 17: 104–16.
3. Galen RS, Gambino SR. Beyond normality: the predictive value and efficiency of medical diagnoses. New York: Wiley, 1975: 129.
4. Manroe BL, Weinberg AG, Rosenfeld CR, Browne R. The neonatal blood cell count in health and disease I: reference values for neutrophilic cells. J Pediatr 1979; 95: 89–98.
5. Zipursky A, Palko J, Milner R, Akenzua GI. The hematology of bacterial infections in premature infants. Pediatrics 1976; 57: 839–53.
6. Tollner U, Pohlandt F. Septicemia in the newborn due to gram-negative bacilli: risk factors, clinical symptoms and hemotologic changes. Eur J Pediatr 1976; 123: 243–54.
7. Schmidt BK, Kirpalani H, Corey M, Low DE, Philip AGS, Ford-Jones EL. Coagulase-negative staphylococci are true pathogens in newborn infants: a cohort study. Pediatr Infect Dis 1987; 6: 1026–30.
8. Christensen RD, Rothstein G, Hill HR, Hall RT. Fatal early-onset group B streptococcal sepsis with normal leucocyte counts. Pediatr Infect Dis 1985; 4: 242–5.
9. Philip AGS. Acute phase proteins in neonatal infection. J Pediatr 1984; 105: 940–2.
10. Sabel KG, Hanson LA. The clinical usefulness of C-reactive protein (CRP) determinations in bacterial meningitis and septicemia in infancy. Acta Paediatr Scand 1974; 63: 381–8.
11. Sabel KG, Wadsworth CL. C-reactive protein (CRP) in early diagnosis of neonatal septicemia. Acta Paediatr Scand 1979; 68: 825–31.
12. Philip AGS. Response of C-reactive protein in neonatal group B streptococcal infection. Pediatr Infect Dis 1985; 4: 145–8.
13. Philip AGS, Andrews PA. Rapid determination of C-reactive protein levels: semi-

quantitative versus quantitative. J Pediatr 1987; 110: 263–5.
14. Ainbender E, Cabatu EE, Guzman DM, Sweet AY. Serum C-reactive protein and problems of the newborn. J Pediatr 1982; 101: 438–40.
15. Philip AGS, Sann L, Bienvenu F. Acute phase proteins in necrotizing enterocolitis. Acta Paediatr Scand 1986; 75: 1032–3.
16. Isaacs D, North J, Lindsell D, Wilkinson AR. Serum acute phase reactants in necrotizing enterocolitis. Acta Paediatr Scand 1987; 76: 923–97.
17. Hanson LA, Jodal U, Sabel KG, Wadsworth CH. The diagnostic value of C-reactive protein. Pediatr Infect Dis 1983; 2: 87–90.
18. Yen-Watson B, Kushner I. Rabbit CRP response to endotoxin administration: dose-response relationships and kinetics. Proc Soc Exp Biol Med 1974; 146: 1132–6.
19. Scheifele DW, Melton P, Whitchelo V. Evaluation of the *Limulus* test for endotoxemia in neonates with suspected sepsis. J Pediatr 1981; 98: 899–903.
20. Togari H, Sugiyama S, Ogino T et al. Interactions of endotoxin with cortisol and acute phase proteins in septic shock neonates. Acta Paediatr Scand 1986; 75: 69–74.
21. Adler SM, Denton RL. The erythrocyte sedimentation rate in the newborn period. J Pediatr 1975; 86: 942–8.
22. Philip AGS, Hewitt JR. Alpha-1-acid glycoprotein in the neonate with and without infection. Biol Neonate 1983; 43: 118–24.
23. Sann L, Bienvenu F, Bienvenu J, Bourgeois J, Bethenod M. Evolution of serum pre-albumin C-reactive protein, and orosomucoid in neonates with bacterial infection. J Pediatr 1984; 105: 977–81.
24. Philip AGS, Hewitt JR. Early diagnosis of neonatal sepsis. Pediatrics 1980; 65: 1036–41.
25 Philip AGS. Detection of neonatal sepsis of late onset. J Am Med Assoc 1982; 247: 489–92.
26. Gerdes JS, Polin RA. Sepsis screen in neonates with evaluation of plasma fibronectin. Pediatr Infect Dis 1987; 6: 433–6.
27. Mathers NJ, Pohlandt F. Diagnostic audit of C-reactive protein in neonatal infction. Eur J Pediatr 1987; 146: 147–51.
28. Edwards MS, Kasper DL, Baker CJ. Rapid diagnosis of type III group B streptococcal meningitis by latex particle agglutination. J Pediatr 1979; 95: 202–5.
29. Bromberger PI, Chandler B, Gezon H, Haddow JE. Rapid detection of neonatal group B streptococcal infections by latex agglutination. J Pediatr 1980; 96: 104–6.
30. Speer ChP, Ninjo A, Gahr M. Elastase-alpha-1-proteinase inhibitor in early diagnosis of neonatal septicemia. J Pediatr 1986; 108: 987–90.
31. Speer ChP, Gahr M, Otte J, Tegtmayer F. Elastase-alpha-1-proteinase inhibitor in neonatal septicemia and hyaline membrane disease. Pediatr Res 1987; 22: 240 (abstract).
32. Okolo AA, Okorodudu A, Glew RH, Omene JA. Decreased serum alpha-amylase levels in infected Nigerian newborn infants. Biol Neonate 1988, 53: 138–43.
33. Mitkowska ZA, Pietrzyk JJ, Pryjma J, Rozanski BS. Chemiluminescence in the diagnosis of neonatal septicemia. Pediatr Res 1987; 22: 240 (abstract).
34. Guillois B, Berthou C, Awad H et al. The importance of C3d estimation in the diagnosis of generalized bacterial infections in newborn infants. Acta Paediatr Scand 1989; 78: 369–72.
35. Sherman MP, Chance KH, Goetzman BW. Gram's stains of tracheal secretions predict neonatal bacteremia. Am J Dis Child 1984; 138: 848–50.

5 Perinatal Listeriosis

J. A. D. Spencer
Institute of Obstetrics and Gynaecology,
Royal Postgraduate Medical School,
University of London and
Queen Charlotte's and Chelsea Hospital, London, UK

Introduction

The name *Listeria* was proposed by Pirie in 1940 (1) for an organism that had two different names in the literature. The microbe had been isolated in England in 1926 (2) following an epidemic of septicaemia in laboratory rabbits; the illness was characterized by large mononuclear cells in the peripheral blood. At the same time, in South Africa, it had been found to be responsible for the death of gerbils with characteristic necrotic foci in the liver (3). Reports of human infection appeared in 1921 and 1929 (4, 5).

Incidence of perinatal listeriosis

Human infections with *Listeria monocytogenes* mainly involve pregnant women and newborn babies (perinatal listeriosis) and the central nervous system of adults, particularly if they are immunologically compromised (6). Perinatal listeriosis was first reported by Burn in 1936 (7) and is now estimated to affect one in 20 000 births in the UK (8). In the Netherlands between the years 1958 and 1977 the rate of listerial infection in neonates and babies under 2 months of age was equivalent to 10 per year (9). Twenty-six per cent of the 424 reports from England, Wales and Scotland between 1983 and 1985 were in children less than 1 month old, and half of these were early neonatal infections (Public Health Laboratory Service, unpublished data). A recent estimate put the rate of spontaneous abortions and stillbirths related to listeriosis at one in 7000 conceptions in the UK (10).

Morphology

Listeria monocytogenes is a short, gram-positive, non-sporeforming, motile rod, whose isolation is enhanced by maintaining a reduced temperature of 20–37 °C. It is also able to grow at temperatures as low as 4 °C, although colonies are not seen for about 10–14 days. Young cultures consist predominantly of coccoid organisms with slightly pointed ends. Organisms may appear singly, in short chains or as pairs attached at one end in a V-shape. It is a facultative anaerobe and there are four antigenic serotypes, of which types 1 and 4 are the predominant ones causing human infection (11–13).

Epidemiology

The epidemiology of listerial infections has remained obscure. Although the organism has

Infection in the Newborn. Edited by J. de Louvois and D. Harvey
©1990 John Wiley & Sons Ltd

been found to infect numerous animal species and has been cultured from soil and faecal specimens, human infection is not primarily a result of direct contact with infected animals (6, 14). There is increasing evidence for transmission by contaminated foods, particularly those kept refrigerated during storage and transport such as coleslaw (15), cheese (16), milk (17) and raw fish (18). *Listeria monocytogenes* may be a normal resident of the intestinal tract but with potentially pathogenic properties; this would explain the widespread prevalence of listeria antibodies among the human population in the absence of clinical disease (6). Rectal carriage by pregnant women was 10 times higher than usual during an epidemic in New Zealand (18). In Israel the symptomless carriage of *L. monocytogenes* in the genital tract was found to be associated with a history of recurrent abortion (19), but this was not confirmed in the UK (20), the USA (21) or Sweden (22). Cross-infection as a source of neonatal infection has been reported (23–25) and outbreaks often occur in clusters (13) or epidemics (26–29).

Maternal illness

A non-specific, influenza-like, pyrexial illness with a cough and headache are the common maternal symptoms of a listeria bacteraemia (30–32), although septicaemia has also been reported (33). Infection in early pregnancy is soon followed by abortion (33, 34), and the degree of maceration at delivery, so soon after the mother's symptoms, suggests that the maternal illness may be a result of, and not the primary cause of, the fetal infection (6). Decidual microabscesses and characteristic foci of purulent villitis within the placenta are highly suggestive of a blood-borne infection with transplacental passage of organisms (35). Severe chorioamnionitis has also been reported, which is in keeping with an ascending pathway of infection (26, 36). Infection later in pregnancy results in preterm labour, associated with meconium-stained liquor (26, 37, 38), stillbirth (32, 39, 40) or an infected newborn baby (41–44). A possible sequence of events is that, following vaginal contamination, the organism infects the decidua and the membranes and may then pass to the placenta itself, where further microabscesses develop. Severe infection results in fetal death, and the process of abortion, or preterm labour with stillbirth, is preceded by release of organisms into the maternal circulation, causing the symptoms described above. Less severe infection results in colonization of the baby at the time of birth, with the possibility of later neonatal listeriosis.

Congenital listeriosis

Infants born with congenital listeria infection following maternal illness are usually also preterm and the labour is characterized by meconium staining of the liquor (37, 38). The usual presenting feature is respiratory distress at, or soon after, birth, but other features include a fever, an erythematous or maculopapular rash, and hepatosplenomegaly (38). Microabscesses and granulomata containing the organism may be found throughout the body, particularly in the lungs, liver and spleen, at necropsy (45), giving rise to the term 'granulomatosis infantiseptica'. The mortality rate of between 35% and 55% reflects the frequency of associated prematurity (26, 27, 38, 46, 47). A high rate of disability among survivors has been reported (38), but this is not always the case (18, 26).

Neonatal listeriosis

Later infection of the neonate with listeria usually presents as septicaemia and meningitis days or even weeks after an uneventful delivery (28, 38, 42, 48–50). The neonates have a normal birthweight and show no evidence of infection at birth. Most reports of late-onset neonatal listeriosis do not include results of maternal investigations, presumably because the infants present some time after birth. Contamination of the genital tract or perineum, or even faecal soiling at delivery, is a possible source of neonatal listeriosis, but has not been firmly established. One confirmed mechanism for neonatal listeriosis is cross-infection by the hands of staff attending either the delivery or the baby subsequently (23–25). The meningitis is a granulomatous macrocytic inflammation of the meninges which may lead on to abscess formation (6). The serotypes responsible are similar to those which cause congenital listeriosis, namely types Ia, Ib and IVb (27). The mortality rate of late-onset neonatal listeriosis is lower than that of the congenital disease (28, 46, 50) and survivors have a low incidence of neurological sequelae at follow-up (38, 50).

Treatment of perinatal listeriosis

Treatment of suspected neonatal infection usually begins prior to bacteriological confirmation. The combination of ampicillin or penicillin together with gentamicin or kanamycin is more effective against listeria than are other agents alone or in combination (28, 51). Listeria septicaemia in the mother during pregnancy has been successfully treated with ampicillin (52), penicillin (53), and ampicillin with gentamicin (43); such treatment prevented perinatal listeriosis. Success in the management of this condition depends not only upon consideration of the diagnosis (54), but on the degree of fetal or neonatal infection at the time of presentation (55).

References

1. Pirie JHH. Change of name for a genus of bacteria. Nature 1940; 145: 264.
2. Murray EGD, Webb RA, Swann MBR. A disease of rabbits characterized by a large mononuclear leucocytosis, caused by a hitherto undescribed bacillus: *Bacterium monocytogenes* (n.sp.). J Path Bact 1926; 29: 407–39.
3. Pirie JHH. A new disease of veld rodents, 'Tiger river disease'. Publ S Afr Inst Med Res 1927; 3: 163–86.
4. Dumont J, Cotoni L. Bacille semblable au bacille du rouget du porc rencontré dans le LCR d'un meningitique. Ann Inst Pasteur 1921; 35: 625–33.
5. Nyfeldt A. Etiologie de la mononucléase infectieuse. Comp Rend Soc Biol 1929; 101: 590–2.
6. Seeliger HPR, Finger H. Listeriosis. In: Remington JS, Klein JO, (eds), Infectious diseases of the fetus and newborn infant. London: WB Saunders, 1976: 333–65.
7. Burn CG. Clinical and pathological features of an infection caused by a new pathogen of the genus *Listerella*. Am J Path 1936; 12: 341–48.
8. McLauchlin J. *Listeria monocytogenes*: recent advances in the taxonomy and epidemiology of listeriosis in humans. J Appl Bact 1987; 63: 1–11.
9. Kampelmacher EH, Van Noorle Jansen LM. Listeriosis in humans and animals in the Netherlands (1958–1977). Zbl Bakt Hyg 1980; 246: 211–27.
10. News. Listeriosis warning too late. Br Med J 1989; 299: 78–9.
11. Larsson S. Epidemiology of listeriosis in Sweden, 1958–1974. Scand J Infect Dis 1979; 11: 47–54.
12. Taylor AG. Listeriosis. Lancet 1980; 1: 1136.
13. McLauchlin J, Audurier A, Taylor AG. Aspects of the epidemiology of human *Listeria monocytogenes* infections in Britain, 1967–1984: the use of serotyping and phage typing. J Med Microbiol 1986; 22: 367–77.
14. Gray ML, Killinger AH. *Listeria monocytogenes* and listeria infections. Bact Rev 1966; 30: 309–82.
15. Schlech WF, Lavigne PM, Bortolussi RA et al. Epidemic listeriosis: evidence for transmission by food. N Engl J Med 1983; 308: 203–6.
16. US Department of Health and Human Services, Public Health Service, Centres for

Disease Control. Listeriosis outbreak associated with Mexican-style cheese, California. Morbidity and Mortality Weekly Report (Atlanta) 1985; 34: 357–9.
17. Fleming DW, Cochi SL, MacDonald KL et al. Pasteurized milk as a vehicle of infection in an outbreak of listeriosis. N Engl J Med 1985; 312: 404–7.
18. Lennon D, Lewis B, Mantell C et al. Epidemic perinatal listeriosis. Pediatr Infect Dis 1984; 3: 30–4.
19. Rappaport F, Rabinovitz M, Toaff R, Krochnik N. Genital listeriosis as a cause of repeated abortion. Lancet 1960; 1: 1273–5.
20. MacNaughton MC. *Listeria monocytogenes* in abortion. Lancet 1962; 2: 484.
21. Ansbacher R, Borchardt KA, Hannegan MW, Boyson WA. Clinical investigation of *Listeria monocytogenes* as a possible cause of human fetal wastage. Am J Obstet Gynecol 1966; 94: 386–90.
22. Ekelund H, Laurell G, Melander S, Olding L, Vahlquist B. Listeria infection in the foetus and the new-born: a clinical, pathological and epidemiological study. Acta Paediatr Scand 962: 51; 698–711.
23. Larsson S, Cederberg A, Ivarsson S, Svanberg L, Cronberg S. *Listeria monocytogenes* causing hospital-acquired enterocolitis and meningitis in newborn infants. Br Med J 1978; 2: 473–4.
24. Campbell AN, Sill PR, Wardle JK. Listeria meningitis acquired by cross-infection in a delivery suite. Lancet 1981; 2: 752–3.
25. Sinha SK, Jones D, Audurier A, Taylor AG. Perinatal listeriosis and hospital cross-infection. Arch Dis Child 1983; 58: 938–9.
26. Becroft DMO, Farmer K, Seddon RJ, Sowden R, Stewart JH, Vines A, Wattie DA. Epidemic listeriosis in the newborn. Br Med J 1971; 3: 747–51.
27. Albritton WL, Wiggins GL, Feeley JC. Neonatal listeriosis: distribution of serotypes in relation to age at onset of disease. J Pediatr 1976; 88: 481–3.
28. Jacobs MR, Stein H, Buqwane A et al. Epidemic listeriosis; report of 14 cases detected in 9 months. S Afr Med J 1978; 54: 389–92.
29. Evans JR, Allen AC, Stinson DA, Bortolussi R, Peddle LJ. Perinatal listeriosis: report of an outbreak. Pediatr Infect Dis 1985; 4: 237–41.
30. Hood M. Listeriosis as an infection of pregnancy manifested in the newborn. Pediatrics 1961; 72: 390–6.
31. Barber M, Okubadejo OA. Maternal and neonatal listeriosis: report of case and brief review of literature of listeriosis in man. Lancet 1965; 2: 735–8.
32. Kelly CS, Gibson JL. Listeriosis as a cause of fetal wastage. Obstet Gynecol 1972; 40: 91–7.
33. Burke D, Ward W, Lucey M. Listeriosis in man. Med J Aust 1973; 1: 292–4.
34. Khong TY, Frappell JM, Steel HM, Stewart CM, Burke M. Perinatal listeriosis. Br J Obstet Gynaecol 1986; 93: 1083–7.
35. Driscoll SG, Gorbach A, Feldman D. Congenital listeriosis: diagnosis from placental studies. Obstet Gynecol 1962; 20: 216–20.
36. Yamazaki K, Price JT, Altshuler G. A placental view of the diagnosis and pathogenesis of congenital listeriosis. Am J Obstet Gynecol 1977; 129: 703–5.
37. Ahlfors CE, Goezman BW, Halsted CC, Sherman MP, Wennberg RP. Neonatal listeriosis. Am J Dis Child 1977; 131: 405–8.
38. Halliday HL, Hirata T. Perinatal listeriosis: a review of twelve patients. Am J Obstet Gynecol 1979; 133: 405–10.
39. Beck A, O'Brian PK, Mackenzie VF. Case of stillbirth due to infection with *Listeria monocytogenes*. J Clin Path 1966; 19: 567–9.
40. Darling MR. *Listeria monocytogenes* infection during pregnancy. J Obstet Gynaecol 1980; 1: 27–8.
41. Johnston WH, Morton SA, Wong MH, Roy TE. Septicemia of the newborn due to *Listeria monocytogenes*. Canad Med Assoc J 1955; 73: 402–5.
42. Harper IA, Howells CHL. Diagnosis of listerial infections in infants. Postgrad Med J 1972; 48: 663–6.
43. Robertson MH, Mussalli NG, Aizad TA, Okaro JM, Banwell GS. Two cases of perinatal listeriosis. Arch Dis Child 1979; 54: 549–62.
44. Barresi JA. *Listeria monocytogenes*: a cause of premature labour and neonatal sepsis. Am J Obstet Gynecol 1980; 136: 410–11.
45. Larsson S, Linell F. Correlations between clinical and postmortem findings in listeriosis. Scand J Infect Dis 1979; 11: 55–8.
46. Ray CG, Wedgwood RJ. Neonatal listeriosis: six case reports and a review of the literature. Pediatrics 1964; 34: 378–92.
47. Relier JP. Listeriosis. J Antimicrob Chemother 1979; 5(suppl A): 51–7.
48. Edmunds PN, Nicholson DN, Douglas DM. Two cases of listerial meningitis in infants. Br Med J 1957; 2: 188–91.

49. Harding JW, Brunton GB. *Listeria monocytogenes* meningitis in neonates. Lancet 1962; 2: 484–6.
50. Visintine AM, Oleske JM, Nahmias AJ. *Listeria monocytogenes* infections in infants and children. Am J Dis Child 1977; 131: 393–7.
51. Gordon RC, Barrett FF, Clark DJ. Influence of several antibiotics, singly and in combination, on the growth of *Listeria monocytogenes*. J Pediatr 1972; 80: 667–70.
52. Hume OS. Maternal *Listeria monocytogenes* septicemia with sparing of the fetus. Obstet Gynecol 1976; 48 (suppl): 33–4.
53. Zervoudakis IA, Cederqvist LL. Effect of *Listeria monocytogenes* septicemia during pregnancy on the offspring. Am J Obstet Gynecol 1977; 129: 465–7.
54. Editorial. Perinatal listeriosis. Lancet 1980; 2: 911.
55. Spencer JAD. Perinatal listeriosis. Br Med J 1987; 295: 349.

6 Perinatal Group B Streptococcal Infections

L. J. Gerards and A. Fleer
Department of Neonatology and Department of Microbiology, Wilhelmina Children's Hospital, Utrecht, The Netherlands

Group B streptococcus (GBS) was not widely appreciated as a potential human pathogen until 1964 (1). In 1887 the organism was recognized by Nocard and Mollereau (2) as a cause of bovine mastitis, and in 1938 Fry (3) described three cases of fatal puerperal infection due to GBS. During this era puerperal fever was mainly due to group A beta-haemolytic streptococci. In 1947 Foley (4) reported 118 cases of human infection caused by streptococci, of which 7% belonged to group B. In 1961 Hood et al. (5) demonstrated the importance of GBS in perinatal and infant infections, and in 1964 Eickhoff et al. (1) reported that GBS was the most frequent single cause of neonatal sepsis during an 18-month observation period in the Boston City Hospital. Over the last 10 years GBS, *Escherichia coli* and *Staphylococcus epidermidis* have become the most common causes of neonatal sepsis and meningitis (6–8). A survey of bacterial isolates from cases of sepsis neonatorum in the neonatal intensive care unit of the Wilhelmina Children's Hospital during a 10-year period revealed that early-onset sepsis was mainly due to GBS (Table 6.1)

During the last 10 years a large body of research has been devoted to the role of host defence in the pathogenesis of neonatal GBS disease. In addition a number of clinical studies have been performed with the aim of improving measures to prevent neonatal GBS disease. Despite these efforts GBS still features as the major cause of early-onset neonatal sepsis.

Table 6.1. *Main bacterial isolates recovered from the blood of 407 cases of neonatal septicaemia admitted to the neonatal intensive care unit of the Wilhelmina Children's Hospital (1977–1986, number of admissions: 2621)*

Isolate	Number of cases	Number of cases: Diagnosed <48 h after birth	Diagnosed >48 h after birth
Staph. epidermidis	166	12	154
Staph. aureus	37	12	24
Group B streptococci	53	38	15
E. coli	65	20	45
Enterobacter spp.	15	1	14

Microbiology

Group B streptococci (*Streptococcus agalactiae*) are members of the genus *Streptococcus*, which belongs to the family Streptococcaceae. The genus *Streptococcus* comprises catalase-negative, aerobic and

Infection in the Newborn. Edited by J. de Louvois and D. Harvey
©1990 John Wiley & Sons Ltd

facultatively anaerobic gram-positive cocci, which characteristically ferment glucose to lactic acid (9). As in all gram-positive bacteria, peptidoglycan (a polymer of *N*-acetylglucosamine and *N*-acetylmuramic acid) is the main cell-wall constituent. The peptidoglycan strands are interconnected by peptide bridges, resulting in a rigid matrix, which not only gives strength to the cell wall, but also serves as an anchoring structure for a number of other constituents, notably carbohydrate units, but also teichoic and lipoteichoic acids and proteins. On the basis of differences in these carbohydrate units a serotyping scheme was developing for haemolytic streptococci by Lancefield in 1933 (10). The Lancefield scheme mainly differentiates between the so-called 'beta-haemolytic streptococci', species which characteristically produce a zone of clear haemolysis around the colonies on blood-agar plates. Species which only produce a greenish discolouration around the colonies are called alpha-haemolytic, and only a few of these, notably group D streptococci, fall within the Lancefield typing scheme. Typically, GBS colonies are relatively large, surrounded by a narrow zone of beta-haemolysis. Group B streptococci are further distinguished by the so-called 'CAMP (Christie, Atkins, Munch-Petersen) reaction' (11). The characteristic feature of this reaction, carried out on a blood-agar plate, is an enlargement by the GBS strain of the zone of haemolysis produced by a beta-haemolytic strain of *Staphylococcus aureus*, when the GBS strain is streaked perpendicularly to, but not touching, the streak of the *Staph. aureus* strain.

Serological identification of GBS is based on a group-specific antigen, a polysaccharide containing rhamnose, galactose and *N*-acetylglucosamine (12). Recent evidence indicates that the group-specific polysaccharide also contains glucitol phosphate (13). However, much more important for human pathology are the type-specific capsular polysaccharides of GBS. Currently, four capsular polysaccharides are recognized, all containing galactose, glucose and *N*-acetylglucosamine, occurring at a molar ratio of 2:1:1 in the Ia, Ib and III capsule, whereas in the type II polysaccharide the ratio is 3:2:1. The structures of these four type-specific capsular polysaccharides were elucidated by Jennings et al. (14–18), and their work has been summarized in a recent review (12). Their studies revealed that all four native capsular polysaccharides contain sialic acid as a terminal residue. In addition it was established that the main differences between the four capsular polysaccharides, apart from the variations in the molar ratio of the component sugars, were determined by the type of linkage of these moieties, both in the polysaccharide backbone and in the side-chain.

The main findings with respect to the composition and structure of the four GBS capsular polysaccharides, based on the studies of Jennings et al. (14–18), are presented in Table 6.2, which also includes data on the major surface-located proteins of GBS, as recently reviewed by Ferrieri (19). The data from this table indicate that the Ic serotype does not really earn this distinction, since it does not contain a type-specific capsular polysaccharide different from the four presented, but it is merely a Ia expressing in addition the c (formerly Ibc) protein. Thus, strictly speaking, in terms of GBS capsular type specificity, Ic is a variant of Ia rather than a separate serotype. Other antigens specific for type Ic have not been detected so far. Serotype II strains also frequently possess the c/Ibc protein (up to 59% of strains), but type III strains rarely do so (5–10% or less) (19, 20). Immune electron microscopic studies using ferritin-labelled conjugates have revealed that the proteins c/Ibc, R and X protrude from the cell wall through the type-specific capsular polysaccharide (21). Thus it appears that, on the surface of GBS, protein and type-specific capsular antigens present themselves in a kind of mosaic pattern, rather than in concentric layers.

Table 6.2. *Major surface antigens of group B streptococci*

*Type-specific capsular polysaccharides**

Ia: →4)β-Glc (1→4) β-Gal (1→ — Backbone
3
↑
1 β-GlcNAc (4←1) β-Gal (3←2) α-NeuNAc — Side-chain

Ib: →4)β-Glc (1→4) β-Gal (1→ — Backbone
3
↑
1 β-GlcNAc (3←1) β-Gal (3←2) α-NeuNAc — Side-chain

Ic: Identical to Ia

II: →4)β-GlcNac (1→3) β-Gal (1→4) β-Glc (1→3) β-Glc (1→2) β-Gal (1→ — Backbone
6 ... 3
↑ ... ↑
1 β-Gal ... 2 α-NeuNAc — Side-groups

III: →4)β-Glc (1→6) β-GlcNAc (1→3) β-Gal — Backbone
4
↑
1 β-Gal (6←2) α-NeuNAc — Side-chain

Surface-located proteins†

c/Ibc:	present on types Ib, Ic, II, III
R:	present on types II and III
X:	not known

Glc, glucose; Gal, galactose; GlcNAc, *N*-acetylglucosamine; NeuNAc, *N*-acetylneuraminic acid (sialic acid).

*Adapted from Kasper et al. (12).
†Adapted from Ferrieri (19).

Based on current evidence it seems likely that virulence factors of GBS are primarily related to the type-specific capsular polysaccharides. In particular, sialic acid, present as a terminal residue on the capsular carbohydrate molecule of all GBS types (12), appears to be associated with a pronounced virulence for newborn infants (22). The relation of sialic acid to virulence may be explained by the fact that this substance prevents activation of complement through the alternative pathway (23), thus interfering with opsonization, which is partially dependent on this pathway. Opsonization through the alternative pathway of complement is considered to be an important part of the non-specific defence system, enabling elimination of microbial and other foreign material when specific antibodies are lacking or the level of such antibodies is low (24), a situation which is often particularly prevalent in the newborn, especially when the infant is preterm (25, 26).

Antibiotic susceptibility

According to *in-vitro* and *in-vivo* studies, penicillin still appears to be the drug of choice in the treatment of neonatal GBS disease. Penicillin tolerance by GBS seems to be uncommon, but may be responsible for a proportion of antibiotic failures. Since it has been documented that combinations of penicillins and aminoglycoside are synergistic towards GBS (27), it may be preferable to treat neonatal GBS disease with such a combination until penicillin tolerance has been excluded. Evidence indicates that some of the newly developed cephalosporins, such as cefotaxime, ceftazidime and ceftriaxone, are very active against GBS *in vitro* and an acceptable alternative to treatment with penicillins (28, 29).

Colonization with GBS in the perinatal period

Among non-pregnant women, rates of colonization with GBS are approximately 4–20% (6). Vaginal colonization is more pronounced during the first half of the menstrual cycle, in women less than 20 years of age and in sexually active women, and is increased in women carrying an intrauterine device. No significant correlation between vaginal colonization with GBS and gynaecological symptoms or the use of oral contraceptives could be demonstrated (30). Male urethral carriage of GBS has also been demonstrated and may occur in approximately 6% of adult men (31).

In the genital tract of pregnant women, GBS colonization rates ranging from 4 to 31% have been reported (31–36). Most data are based on results from single vaginal cultures, taken in the third trimester of pregnacy, or just before delivery. Genital carriage is possibly related to parity. Anthony et al. (37) and Yow et al. (38) reported that the colonization rate was 31% in women with three pregnancies or less, while women with more than three pregnancies had isolation rates of 12% and 18.8% respectively. The differences in carrier rates reported in the various studies may be explained by differences in the culture methods used; the number of different sites cultured; the sites cultured; and the time during pregnancy the samples were taken, since it has been shown that colonization rates may vary during pregnancy (35). Hoogkamp-Korstanje et al. (32) demonstrated, in a longitudinal study of 762 pregnant women, that 75% of all women positive before the 20th week of gestation appeared to be either permanent (59%) or intermittent (16%) carriers. This percentage is much higher than that found by Anthony et al. (35) (36% permanent and 15% intermittent carriers). Hoogkamp-Korstanje et al. also found that 90% of all women positive at labour were positive in the first half of pregnancy (32). This is in agreement with the finding of Ferrieri et al. (33), who reported that carriage was sustained in 81% of women; however, in this study the first cultures were not collected early in pregnancy. In many studies it was demonstrated that the gastrointestinal tract constituted an important reservoir of GBS, and spread to the genital tract may occur from here (32, 33, 35, 36, 39). This may also explain why it is difficult to eradicate the organism with antibiotics.

Serotype analysis of isolates from mother–infant pairs showed nearly 100% concordance, and the transmission rate from GBS-positive mothers to their infant at birth is approximately 50% (32, 33, 40, 41).

In conclusion, neonatal colonization with GBS immediately after birth appears to be the result of vertical transmission.

Persistent carriage and the degree of colonization of the genital tract of the mother at the time of delivery are important determinants for transmission (32, 34). Ancona et al. (34) also showed that the degree of colonization with GBS of infants born to heavily colonized mothers was more intense than that of infants born to lightly colonized mothers. Colonization of a neonate whose mother is positive at delivery appears to be unrelated to maternal age, race, parity or urinary tract infections during pregnancy, to the duration of labour or to the mode of delivery (31, 33,34, 40). Whether preterm are at higher risk for colonization than term infants is unclear.

Up to 40% of newborn infants in hospital may acquire GBS from sources other than the mother's genital tract. Cross-colonization of infants through the hands of nursery personnel may be an important mode of nosocomial transmission (40–43).

Pathology associated with GBS in the perinatal period

Carriage of GBS by pregnant women is associated with maternal and fetal complications during pregnancy. A highly significant increase in the incidence of premature rupture of membranes in women colonized with GBS was reported by Regan et al. (44). Intrauterine death and late spontaneous abortions are also associated with genital GBS carriage; however, the majority of mothers studied were asymptomatic carriers and showed no signs of infection (45–47). Christensen et al. (47, 48) reported that maternal vaginal GBS colonization at the time of labour increased the risk of intrapartum asphyxia, pneumonia and the wet-lung syndrome, compared to the risk to infants born of non-carrier mothers.

Gerards et al. (49) demonstrated that the percentage of small for gestational age (SGA) infants born to permanently GBS-positive mothers was significantly higher than the percentage of SGA infants born to GBS-negative women. The proportion of infants with fetal distress was also significantly higher among infants of GBS-positive mothers.

The most serious disease entities associated with GBS occur in the newborn period, and two clinical syndromes are commonly distinguished: *early-onset disease*, occurring from within a few hours to up to 7 days after birth, and *late-onset disease*, developing after the first week of life. A third type of neonatal GBS disease, also occurring in the immediate postpartum period, was distinguished by Franciosi et al. (31) and called *clinical* or *probable sepsis*. This syndrome, characterized by the clinical picture of early-onset GBS disease, with GBS colonization of skin and mucous membranes, but with negative blood and cerebrospinal fluid cultures, has rarely been mentioned by others.

Infants developing early-onset disease and probable sepsis are generally assumed to have acquired GBS by vertical transmission, either by ascending infection from the vagina to the uterine cavity, or during passage through the birth canal. Perinatal risk factors for early-onset disease are maternal infections during pregnancy and labour, prolonged rupture of amniotic membranes, premature labour, twin pregnacy and a deficiency of transplacentally acquired antibodies (40, 41, 50–53). Early-onset disease usually develops within the first hours of life. The most frequent symptoms are apnoeic attacks, cyanosis, temperature instability and shock; pneumonia is often present. The clinical picture and chest X-ray abnormalities in preterm infants are similar to those observed in idiopathic respiratory-distress syndrome (IRDS), and it is often difficult to distinguish between early-onset GBS disease and IRDS (54, 55). In cases of early-onset disease, blood cultures or cerebrospinal fluid cultures are positive for GBS (31). Early-onset disease is complicated by meningitis in 30% of cases and has a high mortality rate (approximately 50%). The incidence of early-onset GBS disease ranges from 0.3 to 3.7 cases/1000 live births (7, 40, 41, 50, 56).

Infants with late-onset GBS disease, which occurs after the first week of life, may have acquired GBS either by vertical or by horizontal transmission (31, 40). The majority of infants with late-onset disease are severely ill at the time of diagnosis, similar to the infants with early-onset disease; the mortality rate is 20–50%. Up to 70% of the infants with late-onset disease have meningitis (57). The incidence of late-onset disease is estimated to be from 0.3 to 1.7 cases/1000 live births (6, 40–42, 56).

There have been few follow-up studies on infants with neonatal GBS disease. Horn et al. (58) reported that four out of 25 survivors of 44 cases of neonatal GBS infection had neurological sequelae. Wald et al. (59) recently reported the results of a long-term follow-up study of 54 survivors of 74 cases of neonatal GBS meningitis. Sufficiently complete neurological follow-up data were available from 34 infants: major neurological sequelae were present in nine infants, while hydrocephalus developed in another six. These figures emphasize the high morbidity in survivors of neonatal GBS disease.

Role of antibodies and complement in host defence against GBS

From the data collected in epidemiological surveys of GBS carriage by pregnant women, of neonatal acquisition of GBS and of the incidence rate of neonatal GBS disease, it can be estimated that only 1–2% of infants colonized with GBS in the immediate postnatal period actually contract the disease. Evidence has been obtained that the incidence of neonatal GBS disease is significantly higher among infants heavily colonized with GBS than in infants only lightly colonized (41, 60, 61). Together, these data suggest that, in addition to transmission and colonization, there are other factors which determine whether or not GBS disease will occur.

Studies by Hemming et al. (62) and Baker et al. (63) have provided evidence which suggests that opsonization of GBS by type-specific antibodies plays an important role in the protection of GBS-colonized newborn infants against disease. However, the exact role of IgG antibodies and complement in the opsonization of the various GBS serotypes remains controversial.

By employing various well-defined immunoglobulin- and complement-deficient sera, we have determined the opsonic requirements of 14 GBS clinical isolates and five type strains representing all GBS serotypes. The results of these studies are shown in Table 6.3. The data

Table 6.3. *Opsonic requirements of group B streptococci (GBS) in human serum: studies with human pooled serum (HPS), and complement- and antibody-deficient sera*

Opsonic source*	Ia	Ib	Ic	II	III
HPS‡	81.0	74.4	71.2	81.6	79.3
Heated HPS	22.4	9.5	3.9	37.4	5.9
HPS + Mg-EGTA	39.2	19.0	7.8	42.6	23.3
Clq-deficient serum	2.3	5.5	5.3	4.4	3.8
Clq-deficient serum + Clq§	83.0	76.5	62.0	85.3	75.0
C3-deficient serum	22.4	20.5	4.0	61.3	12.7
C3-deficient serum + C3§	65.8	58.3	41.1	83.8	80.0
Factor D-deficient serum	92.8	75.0	72.0	93.3	89.4
Factor D-deficient serum + Mg-EGTA	3.3	8.4	2.1	5.6	3.4
Agammaglobulinaemic serum	5.6	9.9	3.9	14.1	21.8
Agammaglobulinaemic serum + IgG§	78.0	75.0	66.8	82.0	84.6
Agammaglobulinaemic serum + IgG + Mg-EGTA	13.1	7.7	2.4	40.2	6.4

*All sera were tested in a final concentration of 20%, diluted in Hanks' balanced salt solution.

‡Data represent percentage uptake of ^{3}H-thymidine-labelled GBS by normal human polymorphonuclear leucocytes (see Fleer et al. (26) for details of the methods used).

§Clq, C3 and normal IgG were added to undiluted, deficient sera in a final concentration corresponding to the normal serum concentration: Clq, 190 μg/ml; C3, 1300 μg/ml; IgG, 10 mg/ml.

EGTA, ethyleneglycolbis-(aminoethylether)tetra-acetate.

clearly demonstrate that, for optimal opsonization of all GBS serotypes, complement is needed, while activation of complement during opsonization of GBS types primarily occurs through the classical pathway. These observations are in agreement with those of Shigeoka et al. (64), who also found a requirement for classical pathway activation of complement for optimal opsonization of both reference strains and clinical isolates of GBS serotypes Ia, II and III.

A more detailed analysis of opsonic requirements of the various GBS serotypes was performed by Edwards and Baker and their co-workers (65–69). These studies showed that the above findings were indeed valid for opsonization of GBS in control sera, which probably contain only low or moderate levels of type-specific antibodies to GBS. They also documented that opsonization of serotypes Ia and II may proceed in the absence of type-specific antibody and even occurred in the total absence of immunoglobulins, i.e. in agammaglobulinaemic serum, provided the classical pathway of complement was intact. In contrast, we failed to detect any opsonization of the various GBS serotypes, including types Ia and II, in agammaglobulinaemic serum. This opsonic defect was completely corrected by the addition of human IgG, indicating an absolute need for IgG for adequate opsonization of the GBS strains we studied.

Baker et al. (66) showed that, in the presence of a low to moderate concentration of type-specific antibody, optimal opsonization of type Ia GBS may still require an intact classical pathway. However, they also found that opsonization of type II GBS in adult sera containing type-specific antibody may occur through either the classical pathway or the alternative pathway (69). In contrast, in all neonatal sera, opsonization of type II GBS through the alternative pathway was found to be deficient, even in the presence of type-specific antibody. Moreover, some neonatal sera also showed an opsonic defect for type II GBS in the presence of an intact classical pathway, a defect which was corrected by adding adult type-specific antibody at a concentration of more than 2.8 mg/l. A moderate to high level of type-specific antibody either facilitated, or was a prerequisite for, alternative-pathway mediated opsonization of both type Ia and type II strains (66, 67, 69).

Edwards et al. (65) documented an absolute requirement of type-specific antibody for opsonization of type III GBS. As with type Ia, alternative-pathway mediated opsonization proceeded efficiently in the presence of a high level of type-specific antibody, whereas a low level of such antibodies only supported classical pathway opsonization of type III GBS. The authors provided evidence that the terminal sialic acid residues of the type III capsular polysaccharide interfered with alternative-pathway activation, due to binding of the regulatory β1H protein mediated by these residues. The β1H protein promotes rapid decay of C3b, resulting in a decreased amount of this complement opsonin on the bacterial capsule. Fischer et al. (70) and Shigeoka et al. (71) also showed that the amount of sialic acid located on the surface of GBS type III markedly affected opsonic requirements in human serum. In conclusion, these data testify to remarkable differences in opsonic requirements, not only between the various GBS serotypes, but probably also within a single serotype, due to quantitative differences in the composition of the capsular polysaccharides, particularly in the amount of sialic acid.

The role of the surface-located proteins of GBS, notably proteins c, R and X (see Table 6.2), in the pathogenesis of neonatal GBS disease has been relatively neglected so far. A recent review (19) summarized the evidence for the role of protein c/Ibc in providing resistance to opsonophagocytic killing of type II GBS strains. It was found that type II GBS strains expressing the c/Ibc protein were as readily phagocytosed as strains lacking this antigen, but, apparently, the c/Ibc-positive strains resisted intracellular killing (72). In 1975 Lancefield et al. demonstrated protective activity of rabbit antisera possessing antibodies against the c/Ibc protein in mice challenged with c/Ibc-positive GBS strains (73).

The above data also document differences in opsonic activity between individual human sera, partially explained by differences in the level of type-specific antibodies. In addition, the deficient opsonic activity of neonatal serum for type II GBS observed by Baker et al. (69) indicates that the opsonic quality of the IgG molecule after transplacental transfer may be another decisive factor. With regard to this, we have previously demonstrated that opsonic activity of transplacentally derived neonatal IgG for *Staph. epidermidis* (26) and GBS type II (8) is severely diminished. Moreover, we have obtained convincing preliminary evidence that, besides direct opsonic activity, the capacity of transplacentally transferred IgG to activate complement during opsonization of *Staph. epidermidis* and GBS types II and III may also be decreased (74).

The nature of the opsonic defect of IgG after transplacental passage is still unclear; this may be related to structural changes in the IgG molecule induced by the placental transport process, or to differences in the efficiency of transfer of the various IgG subclasses. However, the observed opsonic defect of transplacentally derived IgG towards staphylococci and GBS undoubtedly contributes to the undue susceptibility of the human newborn to these bacteria. Finally, it should be noted that, although it is generally accepted that opsonophagocytosis is an important host defence mechanism against GBS infection, its precise role in protection of the human newborn against GBS disease remains to be defined.

Treatment of neonatal GBS infection

Although, in the future, immunotherapeutic strategies may well become part of the management of neonatal GBS disease, antibiotic therapy will undoubtedly remain a key element of the therapeutic armamentarium. Penicillin continues to be the drug of choice for treatment of neonatal GBS infections, despite reports of tolerance of some GBS strains to penicillin (75).

The combination of either penicillin or amoxicillin with an aminoglycoside such as gentamicin is generally used, since it has been shown that this antibiotic combination may act synergistically on GBS strains (27). For this reason we prefer to start with this combination until GBS tolerance has been excluded and the clinical condition of the infant has improved.

The duration of therapy for GBS septicaemia without focal infection is 14 days. Meningitis due to GBS should be treated for a minimum of 14 days after sterilization of the spinal fluid. Sometimes the dosages of the antibiotics shown in Table 6.4 must be modified to achieve optimal bactericidal concentrations or to prevent toxicity (76).

If GBS should become resistant to penicillin, another antibiotic such as one of the newer cephalosporins, for example cefotaxime or ceftazidime, may be a suitable

Table 6.4. *Antibiotic treatment for group B streptococcal infection of the newborn*

Infection	Duration of therapy (days)	Dosage
Septicaemia	14	Penicillin: 150 000–300 000 IU/kg/day *or* Amoxicillin: 150–200 mg/kg/day + Gentamicin: 5 mg/kg/day
Meningitis	14–28	

alternative (28, 29), although trials to assess clinical efficacy of the newer cephalosporins in neonatal GBS disease are lacking to date. Earlier in this chapter we have discussed the possible role of specific IgG antibody against GBS, of the complement system and of granulocytes in host defence against GBS infection in the neonate. Beneficial effects of blood transfusions, therapy with fresh frozen plasma and administration of immunoglobulins have been reported (77–80). There is, however, a marked variability in the efficacy observed for the various proposed regimens, and randomized controlled studies have not been performed. Moreover, the transfusion of whole blood and the administration of fresh frozen plasma and immunoglobulin preparations is not without risk.

The results of the small number of studies devoted to polymorphonuclear leucocyte (PMN) transfusion in septic neonates appear promising, especially in septic neonates with neutropenia and neutrophil storage pool depletion. Large prospective randomized studies must be carried out before PMN transfusion can be recommended for routine therapy of neonatal sepsis (81, 82).

At the present time therapeutic regimens which may improve the immunological status of the newborn have not found a place in standard therapy.

Prevention of neonatal GBS infection

Colonization with GBS, by vertical transmission, may occur prior to delivery and during passage through the birth canal. This has prompted many investigators to try to prevent or reduce neonatal GBS disease by antibiotic treatment of the mother during pregnancy in an attempt to eradicate GBS from the genital tract, and by administering penicillin to the infant immediately after birth. The earliest studies of antibiotic prophylaxis of neonatal GBS disease were directed towards eradicating GBS colonization in pregnant women during the last trimester (83, 84). In both of these studies colonization was reduced when antibiotics were administered, but re-emerged soon after treatment was discontinued. Merenstein et al. (85) showed a significant reduction in maternal and infant colonization rates when mothers had been treated with penicillin. Treatment started at 38–39 weeks of gestation and continued until delivery. The limitation of this approach is that infants with a gestational age of less than 38 weeks are not treated, yet this group of infants carries the highest risk for the development of serious GBS disease.

Siegel et al. (86) showed a significant reduction both in the prevalence of GBS colonization at 48–72 h after birth and in the incidence of early-onset disease by a single dose of penicillin administered to infants within 1 h of birth. In contrast, Pyati et al. (87) failed to demonstrate any benefit from 100 000 units of penicillin given within 90 min of birth to infants under 2000 g. In most cases of early-onset disease, infection with GBS takes place prior to and during delivery. This supports the view that prevention of early-onset disease must be started prior to delivery. Boyer et al. (88) demonstrated that ampicillin administered selectively during labour to women colonized with GBS resulted in a significant reduction of vertical transmission of GBS to newborn infants. There was also a significant decrease in the degree of neonatal colonization.

Subsequently these authors showed that intrapartum administration of ampicillin to women with positive prenatal cultures for GBS prevented early-onset neonatal GBS disease (89, 90).

Maternal vaccination has been proposed as a possible alternative to prevent neonatal GBS disease (91). However, diminished transplacental transport of IgG in infants born prior to 34 weeks gestation (25, 26) and the fact that some women are low responders to carbohydrate antigens make vaccination a doubtful means of prophylaxis (92).

References

1. Eickhoff TC, Klein JO, Daly AK, Imgall D, Finland M. Neonatal sepsis and other infections due to group B beta-hemolytic streptococci. N Engl J Med 1964; 271: 1221–8.
2. Nocard, Mollereau. Sur une mammite contagieuse des vaches laitières. Annal Inst Pasteur 1887; 1: 109–26.
3. Fry RM. Fatal infections by haemolytic streptococcus group B. Lancet 1938; 1: 199–201.
4. Foley GE. Further observations in the occurrence of streptococci of groups other than A in human infections. N Engl J Med 1947; 237: 809–11.
5. Hood M, Janney A, Dameron G. Beta-hemolytic streptococcus group B associated with problems of the perinatal period. Am J Obstet Gynecol 1961; 82: 809–18.
6. Baker CJ. Summary of the workshop on perinatal infections due to group B streptococcus. J Infect Dis 1977; 136: 137–52.
7. Freedman RM, Ingram DL, Gross I, Ehrenkranz RA, Warshaw JB, Baltimore RS. A half century of neonatal sepsis at Yale. Am J Dis Child 1981; 135: 140–4.
8. Fleer A, Gerards LJ, Pascual A, Verhoef J. Coagulase-negative staphylococcal septicemia in premature neonates: epidemiological features and the role of host defence and bacteriological factors. In: Pulverer G, Quic PG, Peters G (eds) The pathogenicity and clinical significance of coagulase-negative staphylococci. Stuttgart: Gustav-Fisher Verlag, 1987: 215–23.
9. Seibel RH, Seely HW. Streptococcaceae. In: Buchanan RE, Gibbons NE (eds) Bergey's manual of determinative bacteriology. Baltimore: Williams and Wilkins, 1974: 490–547.
10. Lancefield RC. A serological differentiation of human and other groups of hemolytic streptococci. J Exp Med 1933; 57: 571–95.
11. Christie R, Atkins NE, Munch-Petersen E. A note on a lytic phenomenon shown by group B streptococci. Aust J Exp Biol Med Sci 1944; 22: 197–200.
12. Kasper DL, Baker CJ, Jennings HJ. Cell structure and antigenic composition of GBS. In: Christensen KK, Christensen P, Ferrieri P (eds) Neonatal group B streptococcal infections. Basel: Karger, 1985: 90–100.
13. Pritchard DG, Brown GB, Gray BM, Coligan JE. Glucitol is present in the group-specific polysaccharide of group B streptococcus. Curr Microbiol 1981; 5: 283–7.
14. Jennings HJ, Rosell K-G, Kasper DL. Structural determination and serology of the native polysaccharide antigen of type-III group B streptococcus. Can J Biochem 1980; 58: 112–20.
15. Jennings HJ, Rosell K-G, Kasper DL. Structure and serology of the native polysaccharide antigen of type Ia group B streptococcus. Proc Natl Acad Sci USA 1980; 77: 2931–5.
16. Jennings HJ, Lugowski C, Kasper DL. Conformational aspects critical to the immunospecificity of the type-III group B streptococcus. Biochemistry (NY) 1981; 20: 4511–18.
17. Jennings HJ, Katzenellenbogen E, Lugowski C, Kasper DL. Structure of native polysaccharide antigens of type Ia and type Ib group B streptococcus. Biochemistry (NY) 1983; 22: 1258–64.
18. Jennings HJ, Rosell K-G, Katzenellenbogen E, Kasper DL. Structural determination of the capsular polysaccharide of type II group B streptococcus. J Biol Chem 1983; 258: 1793–8.
19. Ferrieri P. Surface-localized protein antigens of group B streptococci. Rev Infect Dis 1988; 10: 5363–6.
20. Bevanger L. The Ibc proteins. In: Christensen KK, Christensen P, Ferrieri P (eds) Neonatal group B streptococcal infections. Basel: Karger, 1985: 101–13.
21. Wagner M, Wagner B. Immunoelectron microscopical demonstration of the cell wall and capsular antigens of GBS. In: Christensen KK, Christensen P, Ferrieri P (eds) Neonatal group B streptococcal infections. Basel: Karger, 1985: 119–27.
22. Baker CJ, Barret FF, Gordon RC, Yow MD. Suppurative meningitis due to streptococci of Lancefield group B: a study of 33 infants. J Pediatr 1973; 82: 724–9.
23. Fearon DT. Regulation by membrane sialic acid of beta 1H-dependent decay-dissociation of amplification C3 convertase of the alternative complement pathway. Proc Natl Acad Sci USA 1978; 75: 1971–5.
24. Fearon DT, Austen KF. The alternative pathway of complement: a system for host

resistance to microbial infection. New Engl J Med 1980; 303: 259–63.
25. Boyer KM, Papierniak CK, Gadzala CA, Parvin JD, Gotoff SP. Transplacental passage of IgG antibody to group B streptococcus serotype Ia. J Pediatr 1984; 104: 618–20.
26. Fleer A, Gerards LJ, Aerts P, Senders RC, Van Dijk H, Verhoef J. Opsonic defence to *Staphylococcus epidermidis* in the premature neonate. J Infect Dis 1985; 152: 930–7.
27. Schauf VA, Deveikis A, Riff L, Serota A. Antibiotic killing kinetics of group B streptococci. J Pediatr 1976; 89: 194–8.
28. Schaad UB. The cephalosporin compounds in severe neonatal infections. Eur J Pediatr 1984; 141: 143–6.
29. de Louvois J. Antibiotics and the neonate: the current choice. Res Clin Forums 1984; 6: 59–68.
30. Baker CJ, Gotoff DK, Alpert S et al. Vaginal colonization with group B streptococci: a study in college women. J Infect Dis 1977; 135: 392–7.
31. Franciosi RA, Knostman JD, Zimmerman RA. Group B streptococcal neonatal and infant infections. J Pediatr 1973; 82: 707–18.
32. Hoogkamp-Korstanje JAA, Gerards LJ, Cats BP. Maternal carriage and neonatal acquisition of group B streptococci. J Infect Dis 1982; 145: 800–3.
33. Ferrieri P, Cleary PP, Seeds AE. Epidemiology of group B streptococcal carriage in pregnant women and newborn infants. J Med Microbiol 1977; 10: 103–14.
34. Ancona RJ, Ferrieri P, Williams PP. Maternal factors that enhance the acquisition of group B streptococci by new-born infants. J Med Microbiol 1980; 13: 273–80.
35. Anthony BF, Eisenstadt R, Carter J, Kim KS, Hobel CJ. Genital and intestinal carriage of group B streptococci during pregnancy. J Infect Dis 1981; 143: 761–6.
36. Dillon HC, Gray E, Pass MA, Gray BM. Anorectal and vaginal carriage of group B streptococci during pregnancy. J Infect Dis 1982; 145: 794–9.
37. Anthony BF, Okada DM, Hobel CJ. Epidemiology of group B streptococcus: longitudinal observations during pregnancy. J Infect Dis 1978; 137: 524–30.
38. Yow MD, Leeds LJ, Thompson PK, Mason EO, Clark DJ, Beachler CW. The natural history of group B streptococcal colonization in the pregnant women and her offspring: I. Colonization studies. Am J Obstet Gynecol 1980; 137: 34–8.
39. Badri MS, Zawaneh S, Cruz AC et al. Rectal colonization with group B streptococcus: relation to vaginal colonization of pregnant women. J Infect Dis 1977; 135: 34–8.
40. Baker CJ, Barret FF. Transmission of group B streptococci among parturient women and their neonates. J Pediatr 1973; 83: 919–25.
41. Pass MA, Gray BM, Khare S, Dillon HC. Prospective studies of group B streptococcal infections in infants. J Pediatr 1979; 95: 437–43.
42. Aber RC, Allen N, Horwell JT, Wilkinson HW, Facklam RR. Nosocomial transmission of group B streptococci. Pediatrics 1976; 58: 346–53.
43. Paredes A, Wong P, Mason EO, Taber LH, Barret FF. Nosocomial transmission of group B streptococci in a newborn nursery. Pediatrics 1977; 59: 679–82.
44. Regan JA, Chao S, James LS. Premature rupture of membranes, premature delivery and group B streptococcal colonization of mothers. Am J Obstet Gynecol 1981; 141: 184–6.
45. Berg T, Hallander HO, Nathorst-Windahl G, Nordlander IM. Group B beta-hemolytic streptococci as an important cause of perinatal mortality. Scand J Infect Dis 1977; 9: 19–22.
46. Bergqvist G, Holmberg G, Rydner T, Vaclavinkova V. Intrauterine death due to infection with group B streptococci. Acta Obstet Gynecol Scand 1978; 57: 127–8.
47. Christensen KK, Christensen P, Hagerstrand I, Linden V, Nordbring F, Svenningsen N. The clinical significance of group B streptococci. J Perinat Med 1982; 10: 133–46.
48. Christensen KK, Dahlander K, Ingemarsson I, Svenningsen N, Christensen P. Relation between maternal urogenital carriage of group B streptococci and postmaturity and intrauterine asphyxia during delivery. Scand J Infect Dis 1980; 12: 271–5.
49. Gerards LJ, Cats BP, Hoogkamp-Korstanje JAA. The influence of group B-streptococcal carriership on pregnancy outcome. J Perinat Med 1982; 10: 279–85.
50. Reid TMS, Hall MA. Perinatal group B streptococcal infection: a 6-year study. In: Parker MT (ed) Pathogenic streptococci. Chertsey, England: Reeds, 1978: 177–8.
51. Pass MA, Khare S, Dillon HC. Twin pregnancies: incidences of group B streptococcal colonization and disease. J Pediatr 1980; 97: 635–7.
52. Edwards MS, Jackson CV, Baker CJ. Increased risk factor of group B streptococcal

disease in twins. J Am Med Assoc 1981; 245: 2044–6.
53. Boyer KM, Gadzala CA, Burd LI, Fisher DE, Paton JB, Gotoff SP. Selective intrapartum chemoprophylaxis of neonatal group B streptococcal early onset disease: I. Epidemiologic rationale. J Infect Dis 1983; 148: 795–801.
54. Katzenstein AL, Davies C, Brande A. Pulmonary changes in neonatal sepsis due to group B beta-hemolytic streptococcus: relation to hyaline membrane disease. J Infect Dis 1976; 133: 430–5.
55. Vollman JH, Smith WL, Bollard ET, Light IJ. Early onset group B streptococcal disease: clinical, roentgenographic and pathologic features. J Pediatr 1976: 89; 199–203.
56. Editorial. Neonatal infection with group B streptococci. Lancet 1981; 2: 181–2.
57. Stringer J, Crees-Morris JA, Young SEJ, Mayon-White RT. Group B streptococcal systemic disease in Great Britain. J Infect 1981; 3: 385–91.
58. Horn KA, Zimmerman RA, Knostman JD, Meyer WT. Neurological sequelae of group B streptococcal neonatal infection. Pediatrics 1974; 53: 501–4.
59. Wald ER, Bergman I, Taylor HG, Chiponis D, Porter C, Kubek K. Long-term outcome of group B streptococcal meningitis. Pediatrics 1986; 77: 217–21.
60. Gerards LJ, Cats BP, Hoogkamp-Korstanje JAA. Early neonatal group B streptococcal disease: degree of colonization as an important determinant. J Infect 1985; 11: 119–24.
61. Dillon HC, Khare S, Gray BM. Group B streptococcal carriage and disease: a 6-year prospective study. J Pediatr 1987; 110: 31–6.
62. Hemming VG, Hall RT, Rhodes PG, Shigeoka AO, Hill HR. Assessment of group B streptococcal opsonins in human and rabbit serum by neutrophil chemiluminescence. J Clin Invest 1976; 58: 1379–87.
63. Baker CJ, Edwards MS, Kasper DL. Role of antibody to native type III polysaccharide of group B streptococcus in infants infection. Pediatrics 1981; 68: 544–9.
64. Shigeoka AO, Hall RT, Hemming VG, Allred CD, Hill HR. Role of antibody and complement in opsonization of group B streptococci. Infect Immun 1978; 21: 34–40.
65. Edwards MA, Nicholson-Weller A, Baker CJ, Kasper DL. The role of specific antibody in alternative complement pathway-mediated opsonophagocytosis of type III, group B streptococcus. J Exp Med 1980; 151: 1275–87.
66. Baker CJ, Edwards NS, Webb BJ, Kasper DL. Antibody-independent classical pathway-mediated opsonophagocytosis of type Ia, group B streptococcus. J Clin Invest 1982; 69: 394–404.
67. Edwards MS, Kasper DL, Nicholson-Weller A, Baker CJ. The role of complement in opsonisation of GBS. In: Christensen KK, Christensen P, Ferrieri P (eds) Neonatal group B streptococcal infections. Basel: Karger, 1985: 170–89.
68. Baker CJ, Webb BJ, Kasper DL, Edwards MS. The role of complement and antibody in opsonophagocytosis of type III group B streptococci. J Infect Dis 1986; 154: 47–54.
69. Baker CJ, Webb BJ, Kasper DL, Edwards MS. The role of complement and antibody in opsonophagocytosis of type II group B streptococci. J Infect Dis 1986; 154: 47–54.
70. Fischer GW, Hunter KW, Wilson HS. Type III group B streptococcal strain differences in susceptibility to opsonisation with human serum. Pediatr Res 1981; 15: 1525–9.
71. Shigeoka AO, Rote HS, Santos JI, Hill HR. Assessment of the virulence factors of group B streptococci: correlation with sialic acid content. J Infect Dis 1983; 147: 857–63.
72. Payne NR, Kim Y, Ferrieri P. Effect of differences in antibody and complement requirements on phagocytic uptake and intracellular killing of 'c' protein-positive and -negative strains of type II group B streptococci. Infect Immun 1987; 55: 1243–51.
73. Lancefield RC, McCarty M. Everly WN. Multiple mouse-protective antibodies directed against group B streptococci: special reference to antibodies effective against protein antigens. J Exp Med 1975; 142: 165–79.
74. Fleer A, Westerdaal NAC, Herngreen S, Timmerman H, Gerards LJ, Roord JJ, Verhoef J. Deficient opsonic activity of neonatal serum: role of bacterial factors and of IgG-dependent complement activation. In: Proceedings of the 4th International Symposium on Infections in the Immunocompromised Host, Ronneby, Sweden, 15–19 June, 1986. Abstract no. 58.
75. Kim KS, Anthony BF. Penicillin tolerance in group B streptococci isolated from infected neonates. J Infect Dis 1981; 144: 411–19.
76. Harris MC, Polin RA. Neonatal septicemia. Pediatr Clin North Am 1983; 30: 243–58.
77. Bortolussi R, Issekutz AC, Barnar DR. The use of plasma infusion for neonatal sepsis. Pediatr Res 1981; 15: 607 (abstract 991).

78. Yoder MC, Polin RA. Immunotherapy of neonatal septicemia. Pediatr Clin North Am 1986; 33: 481–501.
79. Gloser H, Bachmayer H, Helm A. Intravenous immunoglobulin with high activity against group B streptococci. Pediatr Infect Dis 1986; 5: 176–9.
80. Christensen KK, Christensen P. Intravenous gammaglobulin in the treatment of neonatal sepsis with special reference to group B streptococci and pharmacokinetics. Pediatr Infect Dis 1986; 5: 189–92.
81. Cairo MS. Granulocyte transfusions in neonates with presumed sepsis. Pediatrics 1987; 80: 738–40.
82. Krause PJ, Herson VC, Eisenfeld L, Johnson GM. Enhancement of neutrophil function for treatment of neonatal infections. Pediatr Infect Dis 1989; 8: 382–9.
83. Gardner SE, Yow MD, Leds JL, Thompson PK, Mason EO, Clark DJ. Failure of penicillin to eradicate group B streptococcal colonisation in the pregnant women: a couple study. Am J Obstet Gynecol 1979; 135: 1062–5.
84. Hall RT, Barnes W, Krishnan L et al. Antibiotic treatment of parturient women colonized with group B streptococci. Am J Obstet Gynecol 1976; 124: 630–4.
85. Merenstein GB, Todd WA, Brown G, Yost CC, Luzier T. Group B beta-hemolytic streptococcus: randomized controlled treatment study at term. Obstet Gynecol 1980; 55: 315–18.
86. Siegel JD, McCracken GH, Threlkeld N, Depasse BM, Rosenfeld CR. Single-dose penicillin prophylaxis of neonatal group B streptococcal disease: conclusion of a 41 month controlled trial. Lancet 1982; 1: 1426–30.
87. Pyati SP, Pildes RS, Jacobs NM et al. Penicillin in infants weighing two kilograms or less with early-onset group B streptococcal disease. N Engl J Med 1983; 308: 1383–8.
88. Boyer KM, Gadzala CA, Kelly PD, Gotoff SP. Selective intrapartum chemoprophylaxis of neonatal group B streptococcal early onset disease: III. Interruption of mother to infant transmission. J Infect Dis 1983; 148: 810–16.
89. Boyer KM, Gotoff SP. Prevention of early onset neonatal group B streptococcal disease with selective intrapartum chemoprophylaxis. N Engl J Med 1986; 314: 1665–9.
90. Boyer KM, Gotoff SP. Antimicrobial prophylaxis of neonatal group B streptococcal sepsis. Clin Perinat 1988; 15: 831–50.
91. Baker CJ, Kasper DL. Vaccination as a measure for prevention of neonatal GBS infection. In: Christensen KK, Christensen P, Ferrieri P (eds) Neonatal group B streptococcal infections. Basel: Karger, 1985: 281–90.
92. Christensen KK, Christensen P, Lindberg A, Linden V. Mothers of infants with neonatal group B streptococcal septicemia are poor responders to bacterial carbohydrate antigens. Int Arch Allergy Appl Immunol 1982; 67: 7–12.

7 Virological Topics

C. R. Madeley
Department of Clinical Virology,
Royal Victoria Infirmary, Newcastle upon Tyne, UK

Introduction

This chapter is a response to the challenge to say what is new in virology. Perhaps there is little that is genuinely new in virus infections, but we are getting better at recognizing them. The one apparently new infection, by human immunodeficiency virus, is discussed in a separate chapter (Chapter 8), and I have chosen three other topics which have important implications for the newborn. The first involves a recently described virus, the parvovirus B19, although the disease associated with it was described many years ago. Fifth disease has been a disease in search of a cause. Although it is not a major problem, it does cause infection in pregnancy and could induce abnormalities in the fetus.

The second topic is provided by the advent of a drug to treat one of the respiratory viral infections. The predictability and extent of the annual epidemic of respiratory syncytial virus (RSV) merit the term 'Old Faithful', and the appearance of a drug to treat it is an important development.

Third, there are some unanswered queries about virus infections of the gut. It is well recognized that those who are immunocompromised, whether by natural defect or as a result of chemotherapy, are at greater risk from respiratory virus infection. In the particular case of measles, infection may prove rapidly fatal, but other viruses are also capable of doing considerable damage. Surprisingly there seems to be no equivalent vulnerability in the gut and, although fatal infections have been described in immunodeficient children, this is comparatively rare and chemotherapy does not appear to leave the patient at risk. The relevance of this topic to the newborn is that they, too, seem comparatively resistant to gut assaults and this may be related to transferred maternal immunity.

Parvovirus B19

The virus was discovered almost by accident during an investigation into aspects of hepatitis B (1). Although a viraemic stage is present in a number of virus infections, the levels of virus in serum rarely reach levels easily detectable by electron microscopy; this can occur with B19, although its role in causing disease was recognized only about 10 years after its initial discovery. Apart from possible problems in pregnancy, the virus is now known to cause erythema infectiosum ('Fifth disease') (2) and is also a cause of crises in chronic haemolytic anaemias, particularly in sickle-cell disease. An account of human parvovirus infection has been given by Anderson (3).

B19 virus resembles other parvoviruses in structure and in a predilection for infecting rapidly dividing cells. Another member of this group infects puppies, and the clinical disease which follows depends on which cells are

Infection in the Newborn. Edited by J. de Louvois and D. Harvey
©1990 John Wiley & Sons Ltd

developing most rapidly at the time. In newborn babies, in whom the heart is incompletely formed, the virus can cause a rapidly fatal myocarditis, whilst in slightly older animals infected at the time of weaning, or later when there is considerable growth and development of the gut mucosa, the virus causes a haemorrhagic enteritis (4). A similar mechanism is thought to occur with the human virus in patients with a higher than usual turnover of red blood cells. Because the marrow cells are dividing rapidly, the virus finds them suitable for growth, and the consequent infection causes a sharp reduction in new red cell production (5). Because red cell fragility is the underlying problem, the existing red cells are broken down more quickly and a haemolytic crisis develops.

During pregnancy, development of the fetus involves both rapid cellular division and differentiation, giving the virus an opportunity to grow. The delivery of a stillborn hydropic fetus to a woman who had been known to be infected by B19 suggested that this virus could be a problem in pregnancy. Concern that such intrauterine infections could lead to congenitally damaged children has led to two prospective studies, one in the UK by Hall et al. (6) and the other in the USA by Woernle et al. (7).

Hall and her colleagues on the Public Health Laboratory Service (PHLS) Working Party on Fifth Disease have prospectively studied 160 women recruited between January 1985 and March 1987. The women were studied after IgM-class antibody to B19 was found on investigation of a rash or of a contact history in pregnancy. They are or have been followed up throughout the rest of the pregnancy, and subsequently, to monitor the outcome, to confirm fetal infection immediately after birth and to look for evidence of malformation. A sample of fetal tissue or cord blood, and a throat swab and specimen of placenta were collected and examined, as appropriate, for antibody to B19 (IgM or IgG) or for viral antigen by radioimmunoassays, and B19 DNA was detected by dot hybridization using a probe from cloned viral DNA. The babies are being examined as they reach the age of 1 year to assess their general, developmental and serological status. The results to date were reported to the Joint Meeting of the European Society against Virus Diseases and the European Group for Rapid Viral Diagnosis held in Switzerland in September 1987, and are summarized in Table 7.1. It shows the results in 134 women in whom the outcome of pregnancy was known by the beginning of February 1987. Spontaneous abortion or fetal death, the latter usually occurring 4–6 weeks after infection, was found only in the first 18 weeks of pregnancy (Table 7.2). The stage at which infection took place was not known in two patients. In three of the 10 abortuses examined, evidence of B19 viral DNA or antigen (definite in two; equivocal in one) was found. B19-specific IgM antibody was present in two of the 84 cord-blood samples examined and was equivocal in another four. So far no obvious congenital defects have been observed among 15 infants re-examined at the age of 1 year. Immunoglobulin M antibody to B19 was not found in any, but specific IgG antibody was present in four, three of whom had had B19-specific IgM antibody in cord blood.

Preliminary conclusions which can be drawn now are that infection with B19 virus may result in death of the fetus within 4–6 weeks, but does so only in a minority of cases. If the infection does not cause death, however, there is no evidence that the virus leaves any residual damage. Nevertheless, the presence of IgM antibody in cord blood shows that transplacental spread may take place, although only in 10–25% of maternal infections.

It is not yet possible to grow the virus in cell culture, and viral antigen, even for diagnostic serological tests, is in very short supply. Hence there is no immediate prospect

Table 7.1. *Prospective study of human parvovirus B19 infection in pregnancy*

No. recruited into study between 1.1.85 and 10.3.87. All positive for B19 virus IgM antibody	160
No. for whom full information was available	140
No. with rash	128
No. without rash, but positive for arthralgia or 'flu-like' illness	6
No. asymptomatic, but with contact history	6
No. in which outcome is known	134
Live births, with no apparent damage*	109
Spontaneous abortions or fetal deaths	20
Stillbirths	1
Therapeutic abortions	4

*No obvious congenital defects, syndromes or severe abnormalities.

Data from Hall et al. (6) with permission.

Table 7.2. *Virology of parvovirus B19 infection in pregnancy*

(1) Time of fetal death or spontaneous abortion (FD/SA) (4–6 weeks postinfection)

Time of infection	No. infected	No. FD/SA	%
Weeks 1–9	46	7	15
Weeks 10–18	66	11	17
Weeks 19–27	13	0	0
Not known	2	2	—

(2) Direct evidence for infection of abortus

No. examined for DNA/antigen	10
No. positive	2
No. equivocal	1

(3) IgM antibody in cord blood

No. examined	84	
Present	2	7% (Present + Equivocal)
Equivocal	4	

(4) Later re-examination of infants (1 year old)

No. examined	15
IgG antibody present	4*

*Three of these had been positive for IgM in cord blood.

Data from Hall et al. (6) with permission.

of a test for routine surveillance in pregnancy, or of a vaccine. However, the results from this study suggest that infections with the virus will not result in dilemmas over whether or not to terminate a pregnancy. Infection either is lethal for the fetus or leaves no residual damage. While fetal loss will usually be sad for those involved, there is no obvious action to be taken when infection occurs. If it happens in the first half of pregnancy, approximately one woman in seven will lose her baby, but the remaining six should complete the pregnancy and deliver a normal child. However, follow-up of the cases reported by Hall et al. (6) is still at an early stage, and these conclusions may prove to be overoptimistic. Nevertheless, the American study (7), although on smaller numbers, came to the same conclusions.

A virus which probably replicates in rapidly dividing and differentiating cells is in a good position to damage a developing fetus. It will be a few years yet before we can say with complete conviction to an infected mother that, provided she does not lose the baby within the next month and a half, there is little cause for concern. It is essential that tests for B19 infection are made in pregnant women who have an erythematous skin rash (particularly with the 'slapped cheek' appearance of Fifth disease), arthralgia or a haemolytic crisis. Other than counselling, no further action need follow confirmation of the diagnosis, but the child should be very carefully examined following delivery and monitored for the development of more subtle abnormalities as it grows up.

Respiratory syncytial virus and ribavirin

Respiratory syncytial virus is the most common cause of severe lower respiratory tract infection in children under 1 year of age (8). It causes a bronchiolitis from which the majority of babies will recover, provided they are given adequate care, usually in hospital and possibly including the use of oxygen, tube-feeding and active physiotherapy. Infection with RSV is potentially life-threatening, particularly where there are congenital defects in the heart or lungs, and it is recognized to be sufficiently common and severe to warrant developing a vaccine. Apart from the severity, there is a second reason for wanting a vaccine. The virus appears regularly every year and causes an epidemic of sufficient severity to require the admission to hospital of between 200 and 300 babies each winter in North-East England alone. Similar epidemics have been documented in temperate zones throughout the world where adequate diagnostic facilities have existed.

The virus is found also in tropical areas, even where the temperature variations are not so wide. It is capable of causing substantial morbidity, and an experimental vaccine containing formalin-killed virus was produced some years ago. It was discontinued abruptly when it was found that the children to whom it was given were more severely ill later when exposed to natural infection (9). This unexpected finding suggested that hypersensitivity from previous exposure to the virus provided a mechanism by which some children became more ill than others, although it now seems likely that the protective antigens were not present in the vaccine. So far an alternative vaccine has not been developed.

Apart from a very small number of immunocompromised patients, by far the majority of severe RSV infections are in babies under 1 year old. These observations have prompted two questions:

(1) Why is the disease most severe in young babies?
(2) If prevention is difficult or impossible, can the severity of the infection be modified by antiviral chemotherapy?

Part of the answer to the first question may lie in the size of the bronchioles of young babies. The bronchiolar lumen is small and can be more easily clogged by debris following infection. This prevents oxygen reaching the air sacs and hence oxygenation of the blood in the pulmonary capillaries, causing cyanosis and respiratory embarrassment. It is interesting to note that the character of the illness changes as the patient becomes older; in adults, RSV appears to cause nothing worse than a common cold. Because the peak incidence occurs at less than 6 months of age, it can be difficult to find a reliable way of immunizing the child. The solution may be to immunize the mother, although even natural infection does not produce good or lasting immunity in adults. Consequently, the prospect of treating infections caused by this widespread virus with an antiviral drug, ribavirin, has obvious attractions. Trials of the efficacy of ribavirin under double-blind conditions have been reported for several years in infections caused not only by RSV but also by influenza A (10, 11). In half the young adults who had been challenged with virus, there was some evidence of reduction in the time of virus shedding and a marginal improvement in clinical recovery. However, the evidence is not overwhelming and, since the licensing of its use in the UK in November 1987, there is a need to collect further data on its efficacy. As ribavirin is an expensive drug, the obligation to evaluate it properly is strong. The problem is how to do it.

For a variety of reasons, improvements in clinical indices may be slow after disappearance of virus from the nasopharynx, the site from which it is most readily recovered. Table 7.3 lists some possible parameters which can be monitored for evidence of recovery, but in the context of a disease whose natural progress is towards resolution anyway, obtaining verifiable objective evidence of early recovery is not as easy

Table 7.3. *Parameters which could be used to document recovery from respiratory syncytial virus infection*

(1) General
- (a) General impression
- (b) Lethargy
- (c) Poor feeding
- (d) Need for tube-feeding

(2) Respiratory assessment
- (a) Respiratory rate
- (b) Indrawing/respiratory effort
- (c) Accessory muscle involvement (alae nasi, etc.)
- (d) Cyanosis – need for oxygen
- (e) Auscultation
  - Breath sounds
  - Adventitious sounds: wheezing, crackles, moist sounds, etc.
- (f) Quality of respiratory secretions

(3) General assessment
- (a) Pyrexia
- (b) Heart/pulse rate
- (c) 'Restlessness'

(4) Investigations
- (a) General
  - (i) Chest X-ray: Opacity, Hyperinflation, Consolidation
  - (ii) Blood gases
  - (iii) Electrolytes
- (b) Virology
  - (i) Diminished virus production/shedding
  - (ii) Antibody production

as it may appear. Those who have been involved in clinical trials of the drug have usually become convinced that it really does speed recovery, but the evidence they have obtained is marginal. Most have used a clinical score between 0 and +3, extending from complete normality at one end to severe disease at the other. Rather than being derived by a formula, these scores represent an overall impression, that includes the general condition of the baby, the need or otherwise for oxygen or tube-feeding, breath sounds by auscultation, respiratory effort, radiographic appearances and blood bases (if done). Such scores suffer from two defects, both of which are difficult to overcome. The first is that many of these parameters are ways of measuring the same thing and all are likely to improve at the same time, whether recovery is aided or natural. The second is that the short scale leaves little room for clear-cut evidence of improvement. To extend the scale by introducing values for all parameters mentioned is difficult to justify for the reasons mentioned. Nevertheless, Hall et al. (6) have obtained evidence of trends (Fig. 7.1) which suggests improvement without being overwhelming.

Ribavirin is very expensive, with a cost in the region of £200 (US$ 300) per day. This means that it can be offered only to a minority of patients, and the American Academy of Pediatrics (12) has proposed a priority list (Table 7.4). So far ribavirin has only been shown to be effective when given by an aerosol produced by a Small-Particle Aerosol Generator (SPAG) which is essentially a Collinson nebulizer feeding aerosolized drug to a treatment 'chair' with a hood (Fig. 7.2) or, less desirably, to an oxygen tent. The ribavirin is made up as a 20 mg/ml solution in Water for Injection (BP) and given over a period of 18 h. This has been calculated by extrapolation from adult figures and gives approximately 0.86 mg/kg body wt/h. The drug has not been licensed for use intravenously and appears not to be effective orally. As a result the exact dosage given to the patient is difficult to assess, and the method of administering the drug possibly suffers from the serious drawback that mechanical obstruction by cellular debris of the affected bronchioles may prevent the drug reaching the infected areas directly (Fig. 7.2). Ribavirin has been shown to be effective in inhibiting RSV replication *in vitro*, and the

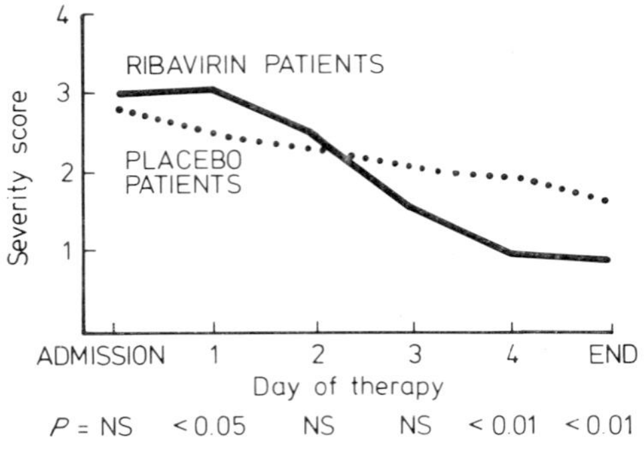

Fig. 7.1. Means of daily scores for severity of illness in respiratory syncytial virus infected patients. A score of 0 is normal and 4 is more severe. Therapy ended at an average of 4.7 days in the placebo group and 4.9 days in the ribavirin group, with ranges of 3 to 6 days. *P* values were determined by the Mann–Whitney U-test and Student's *t*-test. From Hall et al. (10). Reprinted, by permission of The New England Journal of Medicine (vol. 308, pp. 1443–7, 1983).

lack of unequivocal evidence for its efficacy *in vivo* may be due to the difficulties of getting adequate concentrations to the target area.

Expense may prevent routine use of ribavirin in RSV infections in previously healthy children. There is now abundant evidence that the vast majority of these children will recover on adequate supportive measures alone. Rapid techniques of virus diagnosis (13) have ensured that there is less inappropriate use of antibiotics. The use of ribavirin may not shorten time in hospital significantly; hence its use may be confined to severe life-threatening infections which may not be recognized as being dangerous until it is too late for the drug to have any real hope of inhibiting virus replication. These will also be the infections in which all supportive measures will be used and possibly other antiviral therapy such as interferon. Since it would also be unethical to conduct a double-blind trial under these circumstances, it is clear that it will be difficult to obtain further evidence of effectiveness. Nevertheless, continuing evalua-

Table 7.4. *Recommended groups for ribavirin treatment: policy statement by the American Academy of Pediatrics, December 1986*

1. Infants at high risk for severe or complicated RSV infection. This includes infants with congenital heart disease, bronchopulmonary dysplasia and other chronic lung conditions, and certain premature infants. In addition, children with immunodeficiency, especially those with severe combined immunodeficiency disease, recent transplant recipients, and those undergoing chemotherapy for malignancy, should also be considered to be at high risk for complicated RSV infection.

2. Infants hospitalized with RSV lower respiratory tract disease who are severely ill. Since severity of illness is often difficult to judge clinically in infants with RSV infection, determination of the blood gases is often necessary. Infants with PaO_2 levels of less than 65 mmHg and those with increasing $PaCO_2$ levels should be considered as candidates for ribavirin therapy. Oximetry may be used as a non-invasive means of determining the arterial oxygen saturation.

3. Infants who might be considered for treatment are those hospitalized with lower respiratory tract disease which is not initially severe, but who may be at some increased risk of progressing to a more complicated course by virtue of young age (<6 weeks), or in whom prolonged illness might be particularly detrimental to an underlying condition, such as those with multiple congenital anomalies, neurologic or metabolic diseases.

Reproduced from American Academy of Pediatrics Committee on Infectious Diseases (12), by permission of American Academy of Pediatrics, ©1987.

tion should be attempted and we will have to decide how to do it.

Improvement could be measured:

(1) *Virologically*. More rapid disappearance of virus would suggest that the drug was having an effect. However, establishing that this has happened is not as straightforward as it seems. First, it is only feasible to recover virus from the nasopharynx in nasopharyngeal secretions or on a nose and throat swab. The site of significant infection is the bronchiolar mucosa, and disappearance of the virus from the nasopharynx may not parallel disappearance lower down the

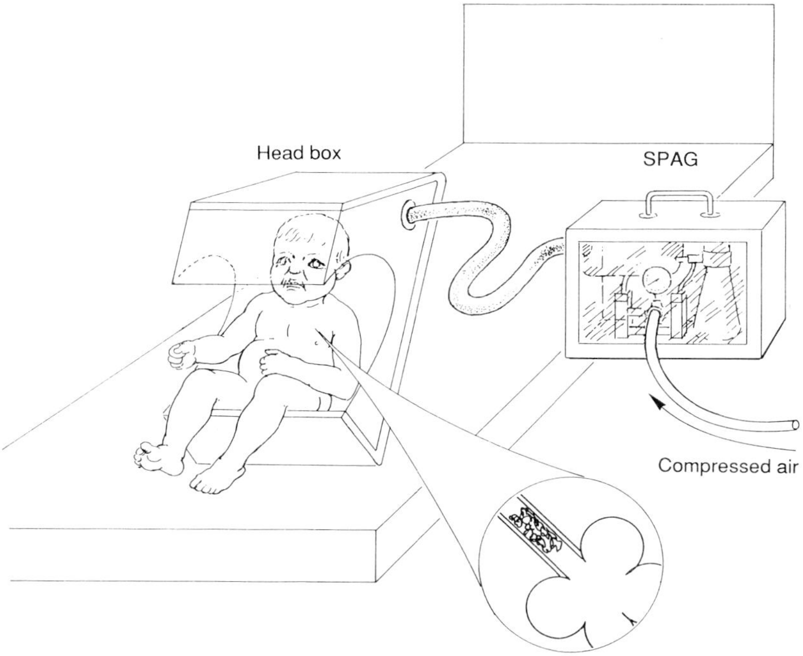

Fig. 7.2. Administration of ribavirin by Small Particle Aerosol Generator (SPAG) into a head box using a supply of compressed air to run the SPAG. The enlarged area indicates partial or complete blockage of bronchioles by cellular and other debris

respiratory tract. Second, quantitation of wild strains of the virus is less easy than of laboratory-adapted strains and also depends very much on the quality of specimen obtained. Poorly taken secretions from the anterior portion of the nose may be seriously deficient in virus compared to the amount present further back. Unless the specimens are taken by a conscientious operator, they are unlikely to be comparable.

(2) *Clinically*. Table 7.3 lists some possible parameters which can be used, but their comparatively slow improvement may mask any true improvement. There are ethical reasons also why repeated chest X-rays and blood-gas analyses should be avoided.

The difficulties of evaluating ribavirin are therefore considerable. Basically, it will mean careful and detailed records of the patient's progress and will probably be handicapped by a shortage of comparable controls. However, long-term follow-up for evidence of permanent damage, as is being carried out in Nottingham by Milner and his colleagues, may indicate the need for more liberal use of ribavirin at the acute stage.

Gut viruses

Until the early 1970s an association between viruses and diarrhoea was assumed but not proven. Studies based on attempts to grow virus showed no clear associations with the viruses which could be grown, and it was only when electron microscopy (EM) was applied directly to faecal extracts that 'new' viruses were found. From 1973 onwards there has been a flood of papers reporting a lengthening list of viruses detected by EM which have been

Table 7.5. *The viruses found in stools*

Groups and members	Number of serotypes	Disease association	Appearance in the electron microscope*	Characteristic appearance[†]	Size (nm)[‡]
(1) *Viruses which will grow routinely in cell culture or newborn mice. Generally well characterized*					
Enteroviruses:					
Poliovirus	3	Poliomyelitis None	Small spherical	No	25
Coxsackievirus A	23	'Poliomyelitis' Aseptic meningitis Encephalitis Herpangina Skin rashes			
Coxsackievirus B	6	Aseptic meningitis Epidemic myalgia Myopericarditis Rashes ?Juvenile diabetes mellitus None			
Echovirus	32	Aseptic meningitis Rashes Non-specific fevers, etc.			
Enterovirus	68–71	?Pneumonia (69) Conjunctivitis (70) CNS infections (71)			
Adenovirus	45	Respiratory tract infections Conjunctivitis ?Gut infections	Large icosahedral	Yes	75
Reovirus	3	None	Large spherical	Yes	72
(2) *Viruses discovered by direct EM. Cannot be grown routinely. Characterization varies from good to virtually nil*					
Norwalk	3?	Epidemic D & V	Small spherical	No	35[§]
Rotavirus	7?	Endemic D & V None	Large sypherical	Yes	78
Astrovirus	5?	Endemic D & V None	Small spherical	Yes	28
Adenovirus[‖]	2	D & V, None	Large icosahedral	Yes	75
Calicivirus	3?	Epidemic D & V Endemic D & V	Small spherical	Yes	35
Small round viruses:					
Wollan or W Ditchling Cockle Parramatta	?	Epidemic D & V	Small spherical	No	22–26
Others[¶]		Endemic D & V			

(*continued*)

Table 7.5. (*continued*)

Groups and members	Number of serotypes	Disease association	Appearance in the electron microscope*	Characteristic appearance†	Size (nm)‡
Small round structured viruses					
Taunton	?	Epidemic D & V	Small spherical	No	30–35
Others¶		Endemic D & V			
Coronaviruses	?	?Diarrhoea	Large enveloped	Yes	100+
		None			
Breda-like	?	?Diarrhoea	Large enveloped	Yes	100+
Others?					
(3) *Bacteriophages*					
Tailed	?	?	Lollipop-shaped	Yes	—
Cubic	?	?	Small spherical	No	20–25

*By negative contrast.
†Appearance in the electron microscope is characteristic, allowing a positive recognition.
‡Approximate size by EM.
§Published size of 27 nm is probably incorrect.
‖Fastidious adenoviruses which do not grow in cell culture.
¶Other similar viruses have been observed from time to time but have not earned individual names.

CNS, central nervous system; EM, electron microscopy; D & V, diarrhoea and vomiting.

Reproduced with permission from Madeley (14).

implicated as causing a gastroenteropathy presenting with diarrhoea, or vomiting, or both. The majority of the patients have been children, but adults have also been involved – mostly in outbreaks.

In the general relief at finding possible culprits for episodes of disease that had been embarrassing the virologists, two apparent paradoxes have been largely overlooked. The first is that the group 2 viruses (Table 7.5), which include those viruses associated with gastrointestinal disease, are not the only viruses which may be recovered from the gut (15). The group 1 viruses, most of which are associated only with disease outside the gut, are frequently isolated from the stools of children with no obvious damage to the gut. These viruses are just as capable of damaging *in vitro* the cells in which they grow, and the paradox is that they do not appear to cause similar damage *in vivo*. In addition, the group 1 viruses are not routinely detected by EM, while the group 2 viruses are only detected because they are excreted at EM-detectable levels. It may therefore be that the former infect fewer cells than the latter. Why this should be so, if the deduction is correct, is not clear, and it means that there is some, presently unknown, factor which limits the spread of the group 1 viruses in the cells of the gut.

The second paradox is that even with group 2 viruses not all such infections lead to overt disease. It is becoming clear that different serotypes of the same virus may have different pathogenic potential, but this is probably not the complete explanation. The relevance to the newborn is that they are less susceptible than older babies to disease induced by group 2 viruses. Several studies in different places have recorded asymptomatic excretion of rotaviruses, astroviruses, adenoviruses and other virus-like particles (16–18).

Several reports have suggested that most infections leading to clinical disease occur between the ages of 6 months and 2 years.

Whether there really is a disease period between these ages is debatable, but asymptomatic excretion, particularly among neonates, has been well documented and none of the group 2 viruses has been recovered exclusively from ill children.

If there is a 'protected zone' in the first few months of life, it is tempting to think that this reflects maternal immunity transferred to the baby. However, there are reasons for doubting this. First, the amount of virus detected in stools of 'normal' children is not clearly less than that found in 'diarrhoeal' children. What sort of protection is this? New virus is produced as a result of infecting virions entering susceptible cells and taking over the intracellular mechanisms, diverting them to the production of virus, and this causes the cells to die. Hence very large numbers of virus particles seen by EM in normal stools should reflect considerable cellular damage, and it seems strange that this is not followed, in turn, by some failure of gut function leading to malabsorption and diarrhoea. Second, the virus particles appear to be devoid of a coating of antibody, which would suggest local production. Even if it were present, although the output virus might be reduced in infectivity as a result, this virus has still been produced in the gut cells, and it is reasonable to expect some evidence of damage. Even in the absence of disease, infection and virus replication to equivalent levels has still taken place.

Perhaps the best example of these paradoxes is provided by adenoviruses, of which there are currently 47 recognized serotypes, with another six candidates awaiting recognition (19). Most have been recovered from faeces at one time or another, but only two serotypes (Nos 40 and 41) have been seriously implicated in causing diarrhoea (20). These are significantly more difficult to grow in routine cell cultures than the others and were not discovered until EM was applied to stool extracts. This led to the intriguing situation

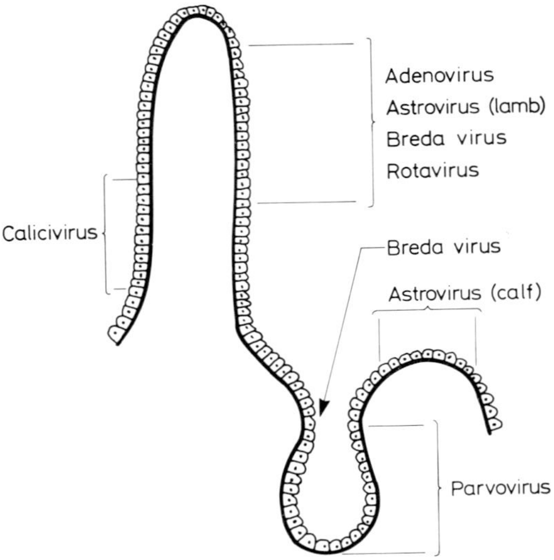

Fig. 7.3. Intestinal villus with preferred sites of replication for various gut viruses. Adapted from Hall (27)

that a stool may have an adenovirus either which can be cultivated but which is not seen by EM (i.e. there is a relatively small amount of virus present) or which can be seen by EM, but fails to grow in cell culture. The more virus present, the more difficult it is to grow.

Experiments in animals and, to a very limited extent, in man have suggested that the group 2 viruses which can produce experimental damage in the gut mucosa are more likely to infect different parts of the intestinal villi or crypts (Fig. 7.3). The cells covering each villus arise from division of the crypt cells and migrate towards the tip of the villus, maturing and differentiating as they go. Individual viruses may prefer to infect cells at particular stages in their development, and this may be due to the expression of appropriate receptors on the surface. At present there is no clear evidence to support this hypothesis, although there has been a suggestion that intestinal lactase may be a receptor for rotavirus (21). Even if this is correct, it does not provide a complete explanation, because what happens is a failure to develop symptoms, not a failure for the virus to replicate.

Further evidence that susceptibility or resistance is not based on immunity is provided by children on immunosuppressive cytotoxic regimens. Respiratory infections which may be very severe are well documented in these children, but gut infections are no more common or severe than in untreated normal children. Interestingly, in both animals and man to whom passive antibody has been administered as pooled gammaglobulin, replication of virus has not been prevented, although the recipients were protected from disease (22–24). The mechanism here is equally difficult to understand.

These paradoxes would not be of more than academic interest were it not for their practical importance in the future. Much time and effort is being put into the development of vaccines against rotaviruses, although not all rotavirus infections are associated with disease. The patchiness in the incidence of disease cannot be dismissed as due to variations in the amount of virus replication, particularly as the levels of virus detected in faeces can reach the order of 10^{12} particles/g. Hence it is difficult to predict how well a vaccine will work in practice. Initial trials in Finland have been encouraging (25, 26), although trials in more overcrowded parts of the world have been less so, and a bovine equivalent did not give satisfactory protection to calves.

Potentiation of resistance may therefore not necessarily involve immunity at all, and an alternative approach might be more appropriate. If so, what should it be?

References

1. Cossart YE, Field AM, Cant B, Widdow D. Parvovirus-like particles in human sera. Lancet 1975; 1: 72–3.
2. Anderson MJ, Lewis E, Kidd IM, Hall SM, Cohen BJ. An outbreak of erythema infectiosum associated with human parvovirus infection. J Hyg 1984; 93: 85–93.
3. Anderson MJ, Human parvoviruses. In: Zuckerman AJ, Banatvala JE, Pattison JR (eds) Principles and practice of clinical virology. Chichester: Wiley, 1987: 507–16.
4. Macartney L, McCandlish IAP, Thompson H, Cornwell HJC. Canine parvovirus enteritis: clinical haematological and pathological features of experimental infection. Vet Rec 1984; 115: 201–10.
5. Serjeant GR, Topley JM, Mason K et al. Outbreak of aplastic crises in sickle cell anaemia associated with parvovirus like agent. Lancet 1981; 2: 595–7.
6. Hall S, Anderson M, Caul EO et al. The outcome of human parvovirus (B19) infection in pregnancy: a prospective study. In: Proceedings of the Joint Meeting of the European Society against Virus Diseases and the European Group for Rapid Viral Diagnosis, Davos, Switzerland, September 1987. Abstract no. S40.
7. Woernle CH, Anderson LJ, Tattersall P, Davison JM. Human parvovirus B19 infection during pregnancy. J Infect Dis 1987; 156: 17–20.
8. Martin AJ, McQuillin J, Gardner PS. Epidemiology of respiratory viral infection among paediatric inpatients over a six-year period in North East England. Lancet 1978; 2: 1035–8.
9. Kapikian AZ, Mitchell RH, Chanock RM, Shvedoff RA, Stewart CE. An epidemiological study of altered clinical reactivity to respiratory syncytial (RS) virus infection in children previously vaccinated with an inactivated RS virus vaccine. Am J Epidemiol 1969; 405–21.
10. Hall CB, McBride JT, Walsh EE et al. Aerosolized ribavirin treatment of infants with respiratory syncytial virus infection: a randomized double-blind study. N Engl J Med 1983; 308: 1443–7.
11. Knight V, McClung HW, Wilson SZ et al. Ribavirin small-particle aerosol treatment of influenza. Lancet 1981; 2: 945–9.
12. American Academy of Pediatrics Committee on Infectious Diseases. Policy statement: ribavirin therapy of respiratory syncytial virus. Pediatrics 1987; 79: 475–8.
13. Gardner PS, McQuillin J. Rapid virus diagnosis: application of fluorescence. 2nd ed. London: Butterworths, 1980.

14. Madeley CR. Viruses associated with acute diarrhoeal disease. In: Zuckerman AJ, Banatvala JE, Pattison JR (eds) Principles and practice of clinical virology. Chichester: Wiley, 1987: 159–96.
15. Madeley CR. Viruses in the stools. J Clin Pathol 1979; 32: 1–10.
16. Chrystie IL, Totterdell BM, Banatvala JE. Asymptomatic endemic rotavirus infections in the newborn. Lancet 1978; 1: 1176–8.
17. Murphy AM, Albrey MB, Crewe EB. Rotavirus infections of neonates. Lancet 1977; 2: 1149–50.
18. Cameron DJS, Bishop RF, Veenstra AA et al. Pattern of shedding of two noncultivatable viruses in stools of newborn babies. J Med Virol 1978; 2: 7–13.
19. Hierholzer JC, Wigand R, Anderson LJ et al. Adenovirus from patients with AIDS. J Infect Dis 1988; 158: 804–13.
20. Uhnoo I, Wadell G, Svensson L, Johansson M. Two new serotypes of enteric adenovirus causing infantile diarrhoea. Develop Biol Stand 1983; 53: 311–18.
21. Holmes IH, Rodger SM, Schnagl RD et al. Is lactose the receptor and uncoating enzyme for infantile enteritis (rota) viruses? Lancet 1976; 1: 1387–8.
22. Snodgrass DR, Wells PW. Rotavirus infection in lambs: studies on passive protection. Arch Virol 1976; 52: 201–5.
23. Snodgrass DR, Madeley CR, Wells PW, Angus KW. Human rotavirus in lambs: infection and passive protection. Infect Immun 1977; 16: 268–70.
24. Barnes GL, Doyle LW, Hewson PH et al. A randomised trial of oral gamma globulin in low-birth-weight infants infected with rotavirus. Lancet 1982; 1: 1371–3.
25. Vesikari T, Isolauri E, Delem A, D'Hondt E, Andre FE, Zissis G. Immunogenicity and safety of live oral attenuated bovine rotavirus vaccine strain RIT 4237 in adults and young children. Lancet 1983; 2: 807–11.
26. Vesikari T, Isolauri E, D'Hondt E, Delem A, Andre FE, Zissis G. Protection of infants against rotavirus diarrhoea by RIT 4237 attenuated bovine rotavirus strain vaccine. Lancet 1984; 1: 977–81.
27. Hall GA. Comparative pathology of infection by novel diarrhoeal viruses. In: Bock G, Whelan J (eds) Novel diarrhoeal viruses. CIBA Foundation Symposium, no. 128. Chichester: Wiley, 1987: 192–207.

8 Practical Aspects of Human Immunodeficiency Virus Infection in the Newborn

C. Giaquinto, A. de Rossi, R. d'Elia,
L. Chieco-Bianchi and F. Zacchello
Department of Paediatrics and Institute of Oncology, University of Padova, Italy

Paediatric acquired immunodeficiency syndrome (AIDS) was first described in 1982, when a child with opportunistic infection was reported (1). By December 1988, 1346 children with AIDS had been reported to the US Centers for Disease Control (CDC) (2). Some of these patients had received blood transfusions, but 80% were born to human immunodeficiency virus (HIV) seropositive mothers belonging to high-risk groups for AIDS. In Italy the prevalence of HIV infection among intravenous drug users (IVDUs) ranges from 40 to 80% in different urban areas, and is higher than in most European countries (3). There is clear evidence that the infection in infants can be acquired transplacentally from the mother (4), but there are insufficient data to confirm whether infection may be acquired during delivery (5) or from breast milk (6). The definition of paediatric AIDS unfortunately is limited and does not cover important aspects of symptomatic HIV infection in childhood (7); however, in Italy, children with full-blown AIDS represent 3% of all reported cases (8). Moreover, by March 1990 more than 1300 seropositive children had been reported to the Italian Registry of Paediatric HIV Infection (P.A. Tovo, personal communications); it is estimated that this number will increase in the next 5 years due to the increasing number of women of childbearing age who become infected.

The number of children alone does not reflect the impact of paediatric AIDS on the population. The total dependence of young children and the fact that most HIV-infected children are sick from infancy mean that entire families are struggling, from the babies' birth, with the tragic and constantly shifting course of the infection. Most of the children have parents with drug-abuse problems (2) that may seriously affect their ability to meet this enormous responsibility; it is also not infrequent for other family members to be suffering from AIDS.

In 1985 the Department of Paediatrics and the Institute of Oncology of the University of Padova undertook a multidisciplinary programme on paediatric AIDS (9). The main goals of this project were to assist HIV-infected children and their families and to study the natural history of the infection with the European collaborative study group (4, 10). Our working study group includes paediatricians, obstetricians, child psychiatrists, virologists, immunologists, social workers and a coroner. To date, all the children studied (150) acquired the infection from their mothers (95% IVDUs), probably *in utero* (11).

Infection in the Newborn. Edited by J. de Louvois and D. Harvey
©1990 John Wiley & Sons Ltd

During our work, questions were raised about many aspects of the clinical management of pregnancy and the neonatal period. Although numerous critical questions remain unanswered, this paper will review our experiences and our guidelines on some practical aspects of HIV infection in pregnant women and their children.

Antenatal HIV screening and management of seropositive women

The existence of HIV-antibody screening tests, and their use in many countries on blood from donors, has raised questions as to whether low-risk groups (such as military recruits, pregnant women or health-care workers) should be screened (11). In 1987 the Istituto Superiore di Sanità (8) produced a study on a hypothetical generalized screening of pregnant women in Italy, where there are about 700 000 deliveries per year. Assuming that this approximates to the number of pregnant women and that the prevalence is 1/20 000, it was estimated that about 34 infected women would be identified per year. Since screening tests (ELISA) have a sensitivity of 99% and an 'operative' specificity of 95%, universal screening would result in about 35 000 false-positive tests (positive predictive value 0.001), which would require further tests (Western blot) to confirm the diagnosis of infection. The cost of identifying each positive woman would be about 420 000 000 Italian lire (UK sterling 200 000).

A more realistic analysis, considering the higher prevalence of HIV infection in women of childbearing age (5/1000) and an ELISA specificity of 98%, also results in 14 000 false-positive tests (positive predictive value 0.09) (Table 8.1) (12) The presence of so many 'false-positive' women at the first test would make such screening in pregnancy dangerous, because of the great anxiety which would be caused and the high rate of useless terminations which would occur.

When we started to study perinatal HIV transmission in Padova in 1985, our first problem was how to identify infected pregnant women. To estimate the prevalence of the infection, we screened 360 women after

Table 8.1. *Estimated results of yearly human immunodeficiency virus (HIV) screening of all pregnant women in Italy*

Assuming:
- -100 000–150 000 seropositive persons (25–30% women, most 18–33 years old)
- 6 000 000 women 18–33 years old
  - -*5/1000* prevalence of HIV infection in women aged 18–33 years in Italy
- Fertility rate 5%
  - -*1500* pregnancies/year in seropositive women in Italy (5% of 30 000 estimated seropositive women)
- -Screening test (ELISA) specificity 98%
  sensitivity 99%

Test	Infected	Not infected	Total
Positive	1485	13 970	15 455
Negative	15	684 530	684 545
Total	1500	698 500	700 000

Positive predictive value 0.09.
Negative predictive value 0.9999.

informed consent at the time of delivery. Twenty-three were positive by ELISA, but only two, both IVDUs, were confirmed by Western blot. Therefore we decided to screen only women at high risk of being infected: IVDUs (present or past), blood-transfusion recipients (after 1979), HbsAg-positive women from countries with high prevalence of HIV and those with partners in 'risk' groups. Hepatitis B is common in Italy, particularly among IVDUs, so we thought that by using this marker we would be able to detect some positive women. This screening is carried out by neonatal clinics or at the time of delivery.

In order to discover whether the infection had spread from the above 'risk' groups to the general population, we screened 277 pregnant women in 1987. One of them was seropositive and she was an IVDU.

Plans to test low-risk populations for HIV antibodies generally ignore the risk of false-positive results. These mistakes may change the lives of people who are incorrectly identified as infected – couples, for example, remaining childless to avert the birth of a child with AIDS (13). When screening of blood donors began in 1985, decontaminating the blood supply was an urgent need. But before we establish a public policy of widespread screening, we should consider whether what is justified in the blood blank is also justified in other settings. Unless the false-positive rate of screening tests is virtually zero, the screening of pregnant women in whom the prevalence of HIV is low will unavoidably stigmatize and frighten many healthy people.

All women with high-risk factors should be offered an HIV-antibody test before becoming pregnant or when pregnant. Depending on the prevalence of HIV infection in a country, the availability of laboratory facilities and cost–benefit analysis, the test may be considered for all pregnant women. All women found to be HIV positive or with high-risk factors must be offered, together with their partners, good counselling and educational advice on a personal and confidential basis. This must include information about the implications of the infection for the pregnancy and the newborn infant.

In countries where termination of pregnancy is acceptable it should be offered at an early stage to all women known to be HIV positive or at continuing risk of exposure to HIV infection (such as drug addicts, partners of seropositive men, etc). The justification for this is to prevent the birth of an HIV-infected infant; the view that pregnancy can accelerate HIV disease is not confirmed by prospective studies (14). However, the final decision must be left to the women, who may also decide to take the chance of having an uninfected child. In our experience among many past drug users the psychological and social importance of having a child far exceed the risk of having an infected baby.

Since at present there is no prenatal diagnosis, counselling and education of seropositive women who decide to continue pregnancy must be offered regularly. Confidentiality must be ensured to minimize the risk that HIV-infected women and their children will be subject to discrimination.

Mode of delivery

The most important mode of transmission of HIV infection from mother to child is intrauterine (4). In addition, HIV has been isolated from cervical secretions, which suggests that these could be another source of infection (15). In 1986 Chiodo *et al.* described 12 infants born to HIV-positive mothers and followed up for 6–12 months (5). All mothers showed immunological abnormalities and five had AIDS-related conditions (ARC). Three of the seven infants born by vaginal delivery had HIV antibodies – a difference that is not statistically significant. The authors recommended delivery by caesarian section for HIV-positive women, but their data are far from conclusive, particularly in view of the higher proportion with ARC in the vaginal delivery group (4/7 vs 1/5). Moreover, the diagnosis of infection was made only on the basis of the presence of HIV-specific antibody, which if passively transferred could even disappear after 18 months of age.

Using the CDC criteria for diagnosis of paediatric HIV infection (16), we studied the outcome of 55 pregnancies (36 by vaginal delivery and 19 by caesarian section) Table 8.2). Thirteen out of 36 children born by vaginal delivery were infected versus seven out of 19 born by caesarian section. The difference was not statistically significant.

Several prospective studies have evaluated the risk of HIV transmission by vaginal delivery (10, 17). These suggest that mode of delivery does not influence transmission rate, but the small sample size and other confounding variables made accurate risk estimates impossible.

To date there is inadequate evidence to support the view that caesarian section reduces the risk of HIV transmission to the newborn, and caesarian section carries some maternal and neonatal risks which may be enhanced in a potentially immunocompromised individual. Therefore, comparing the hazards and the benefits of such an approach, it is our opinion that caesarian section should not be mandatory on the basis of maternal HIV infection alone.

Breast-feeding

The possibility that HIV infection could be transmitted by breast-feeding was raised by the isolation of HIV from the acellular fraction of breast milk of healthy carriers (18). The first case report in 1985 concerned a child whose mother presumably seroconverted following caesarian section, after receiving a blood transfusion from a donor who was later found to have AIDS. The baby was breast-fed for 6 weeks and when the first serological tests were done, at 18 months, both the child and the mother were found to be positive, while the father and older children were negative (6).

Table 8.2. *Relation between mode of delivery and infection*

	Infected	Not infected	Total
Vaginal	13	23	36
Caesarian section	7	12	19
Total	20	35	55

Differences are not significant.

On the basis of these reports a breast-feeding policy, formulated in 1985 by the CDC, suggests that 'HTLV-III/LAV infected women should be advised against breast feeding to avoid postnatal transmission to a child who may not be infected' (19).

To date, few further cases ($n = 9$) have been reported. In all but one the mother was thought to have been infected just after pregnancy by postnatal blood transfusion (seven cases) or needle-sharing (one case). The other child, born in Zaire, developed AIDS after being breast-fed since birth by an HIV-positive wet nurse with ARC; no clinical and laboratory data were available on the natural mother or on the wet nurse (20).

Even though we would consider these as proven cases of breast-milk transmission, all but one of the children were breast-fed by their mothers soon after the acquisition of HIV. This does not necessarily imply that such transmission occurs in mothers who were HIV infected before or during pregnancy. Newly infected persons as well as those with advanced immunodeficiency have higher titres of circulating virus and a higher proportion of infected lymphocytes and may be more infectious. Moreover, infants breast-fed by mothers infected after delivery are exposed to HIV in the absence of pre-existing maternal antibody, which could have some protective effect.

Seventeen out of 271 babies enrolled in the European Collaborative Study (10, 21) were breast-fed from 1 week to 7 months; ten are considered to be free from infection (seronegative, virus- and/or antigen-negative; no symptoms), four are indeterminate (16) and three are infected. Two of them have AIDS and clinical symptoms appeared in the first 2 months of life, suggesting that both infants were infected *in utero*. At least 10 out of 17 breast-fed babies are apparently not infected and, although these numbers are too small to allow a conclusion to be reached, they do add to the impression that breast-feeding is not a common source of infection.

To demonstrate the relative risk of infection in breast-fed children, 102 children born to seropositive mothers were prospectively evaluated for more than 2 years in Zaire. It was found that 20% of breast-fed and 19% of formula-fed infants were infected; the difference was not significant. The authors concluded that in Africa all mothers should breast-feed their children until weaning (22).

To date, the risk of HIV transmission from mother to infant through breast milk has not been well defined. Although it seems reasonable to believe that breast-feeding during seroconversion carries a relatively high risk of transmission of HIV infection, breast-feeding after a seropositive pregnancy may not involve any additional risks. However, the importance of co-factors, the prognostic values of antigen and virus testing on maternal blood or colostrum remain unknown; it is still unclear if continuous exposure to HIV through breast-feeding in already infected children may affect the course of the infection.

The situation certainly needs further investigation, but we have to deal daily with questions regarding the advice which should be given to HIV-positive mothers on breast-feeding. We need a clear answer, whereas guidelines given by the CDC, the Department of Health and Social Security (DHSS), and the World Health Organization (WHO) are far from concordant.

The unique immunological, nutritional and psychosocial benefits of breast milk are well known. In HIV-infected children maternal milk is also important in preventing intercurrent infection which could accelerate the course of disease. We must balance the potential benefits of breast-feeding in each country with the additional theoretical risk of infection to the infant born to the HIV-positive mother. Consideration should be given to the socioeconomic and ecological environment of the mother–child pair and the extent to which alternative methods of feeding can safely and effectively be used. Since the balance of risk is different in developing and developed countries, guidelines must take into account the different conditions.

Guidelines for advice on breast-feeding

The mother who is considered to be infected should be advised of the possible additional risk of infecting her babies through breast-feeding but should be discouraged from doing so only when alternative methods of feeding are safe and effective (adequate breast-milk substitute, clean water for dilution, refrigeration, etc.).

In some developing countries, despite the high prevalance of HIV infection in the population and the risk of maternal seroconversion during breast-feeding, the importance of breast milk for the survival and development of infants needs no explanation. Breast-feeding by the biological mother should continue to be the feeding method of choice, regardless of her HIV infectious status.

Seronegative mothers who are at continuing risk of exposure to HIV infection (drug addicts, partners of seropositive men, etc.) should be serologically evaluated during pregnancy and should be counselled about the importance of avoiding risk behaviours.

If a woman continues to be exposed to the risk of infection, she should be informed of the additional risk of breast-feeding for her baby.

Further advice should be given on an individual basis. When there is strong evidence suggesting that the woman might be infected, although still seronegative at the end of pregnancy, she should be discouraged from breast-feeding if there are valid alternatives.

When an infected or 'at-risk' mother breast-feeds, she should continue to receive appropriate care for herself and the infant. If she is treated with antiretroviral drugs, special attention should be given to the possible side-effect of the drug to the baby.

Milk banking

In many countries pooled breast milk is used in certain circumstances, such as to feed premature babies, after neonatal surgery and in severe cases of cow's milk intolerance (23, 24). There is a debate as to whether or not to close human milk banks on the grounds that infants might contract HIV infection from infected donors (25).

Since a policy of compulsory screening of donors might reduce the number of volunteers, the pasteurization of pooled milk was evaluated (26). Two commercial pasteurization systems were found to inactivate virus infectivity at a level which greatly exceeded that found naturally in one donation of breast milk. The authors concluded that pasteurization of pooled milk eliminates the risk of HIV transmission and that HIV-antibody screening of donors is therefore unnecessary. However, concerns were expressed by others about the susceptibility of cell-free HIV to pasteurization (27). Considering that pasteurization alone could not eliminate the theoretical risk of infection, the DHSS recommended in 1988 that donors of breast milk should be tested for HIV monthly, with cryostorage of donated milk for 3 months until it was certain that donors were HIV negative.

As the positive predictive value of HIV screening tests is relatively low in populations with a low prevalence of infection, such as milk donors, we think that this policy would create a great deal of needless anxiety in uninfected women (due to false-positive results) and would discourage them from donating milk. Women who are seropositive or who are at continuing risk of exposure should have been identified during pregnancy and should not donate milk. If guidelines for identification of such women have been followed, there is no need for additional screening.

All donors must be carefully informed (by the use of questionnaires or leaflets) about the dangers of 'at-risk' women donating milk and the importance of HIV testing. However, all donated milk should be pasteurized, even if this alone cannot be relied upon as an infallible method for preventing HIV transmission.

The possibility of screening donors should be considered in areas where the prevalence of HIV infection is known to be high. Similarly, if for some reason the natural mother cannot breast-feed and wet-nursing is the next obvious method of choice the risk of HIV infection should be borne in mind.

Immunization

The immunological abnormalities associated with HIV infection have given rise to concern about the immunization of seropositive children (28–30). The replication of live attenuated vaccine virus may be enhanced in these patients, as in children with primary immunodeficiency, and may produce serious adverse effects. Concern has been expressed also about the theoretical risk that repeated antigenic stimulation, such as that by live or inactivated vaccines, might accelerate the course of the infection (31).

Live vaccines are usually contraindicated in children with immunodeficiencies because of the potential risk of disseminated infection with the viral or bacterial vaccine strain (32). However, HIV-infected children are not always immunodeficient, as there is a period when their immune system is not compromised

(33). Assessment of live-vaccine safety is complicated by the fact that it is not always clear whether HIV-infected patients are immunodeficient or not at the time of immunization. Moreover, although inactivated vaccines are not usually contraindicated in patients with immunodeficiency, some concern has been expressed about the risk of accelerating the course of HIV infection with repeated antigenic stimulation (33).

A case was described of a military recruit with asymptomatic HIV who became symptomatic and developed disseminated vaccinia infection after receiving the customary battery of immunization during basic training (31). *In-vitro* studies have shown that the activation of HIV-infected lymphocytes leads to HIV expression followed by cell death, suggesting that repeated antigenic stimulation might precipitate the development of AIDS (34).

To evaluate this effect *in vivo*, a cohort of seropositive homosexual or bisexual men were randomized to receive hepatitis B vaccine or placebo. There was no difference in the prevalence of AIDS/ARC in the two groups (35). Another study indicated that hepatitis B vaccination in seropositive men has no detrimental effect on the CD4 cell count (36).

In order to examine the safety of routine immunization the New York City Department of Health conducted a retrospective survey on 188 children who received a total of 468 doses of live oral poliovirus vaccine (OPV) and 70 children who received measles, mumps and rubella virus vaccine (MMR) or measles vaccine. No adverse events were reported (30). Several prospective studies in Europe and Africa have failed to demonstrate any serious adverse reaction to OPV, inactivated poliovirus vaccine (IPV), diphtheria and tetanus toxoids and pertussis vaccine (DTP), MMR and measles vaccine (10, 17, 37, 38).

The maximal theoretical risk of serious adverse events occurring following immunization has been estimated from retrospective and prospective studies (30). For OPV, based on over 400 HIV-infected vaccinated children, the maximal theoretical risk is 0.8%; for MMR or measles vaccine, 1.4%.

The only complications following administration of live vaccine were reported in France, where five children developed local lymphadenitis after receiving bacille Calmette-Guérin vaccine (BCG) (39). However, HIV-infected and uninfected control children, followed prospectively in Zaire and Kenya, had similar rates of regional lymphadenitis and fever following BCG vaccination (38–40).

Human immunodeficiency virus infection in children produces both cellular and humoral immunodeficiency (41). Immunological dysfunctions range from no obvious deficit to severe combined immunodeficiency. Data on immunogenicity in children show that both primary and secondary antibody responses are reduced, especially in symptomatic patients (42). Studies on antibody response to different types of vaccine are reported in Table 8.3.

Children with symptomatic HIV infection have lower serum concentrations of diphtheria, tetanus and measles antibodies than have age-matched controls. Nevertheless, substantial proportions of HIV-infected children respond with serum antibody concentrations considered protective. These findings suggest that there is a potential benefit to immunizing HIV-infected children before their immune systems are further compromised. The serological response to several vaccines is inversely correlated to the severity of symptoms associated with HIV infection (33). However, from these studies it seems reasonable to conclude that immunizing children early in the course of HIV infection might be beneficial in reducing the subsequent increased risk of infections observed in advanced cases of HIV disease.

Epidemiological considerations of the incidence of vaccine-target diseases are needed before establishing any immunization policy. Most information available relates to measles. Studies conducted in the USA and Africa have shown that the case-fatality rate during acute

Table 8.3. *Vaccine immunogenicity in children infected with human immunodeficiency virus*

Country*	Type of vaccine	No. of children studied (AIDS/ARC)†	% antibody response	
			Infected	Control
USA (43)	Measles	10	60	
USA (44)	OPV	23	91	
USA (44)	IPV	3	100	
France (39)	DTP	7 (7)	57‡	
France (39)	DTP	13 (13)	61§	
USA (45)	DTP	17 (17)	17§	100
USA (45)	DTP	17 (15)	60§	100
Italy‖	DT/DTP	12 (4)	100§	
USA (46)	OPV/IPV	29	90/100	
USA (46)	Measles	23	39	
USA (46)	Mumps	23	19	
USA (46)	Rubella	23	45	

*References to studies are given in parentheses.
†Numbers of children with AIDS/ARC given in parentheses.
‡Serological response to diphtheria toxoid.
§Serological response to tetanus toxoid.
‖Unpublished data.

AIDS, acquired immunodeficiency syndrome; ARC, AIDS-related conditions; OPV, live oral poliovirus vaccine; IPV, inactivated poliovirus vaccine; DTP, diphtheria and tetanus toxoids and pertussis vaccine.

measles was significantly higher in HIV-infected children than in uninfected children (30, 37).

There have been no reports of poliomyelitis, diphtheria or tetanus in HIV-infected persons. Pertussis cases, including one reported death (47), have occurred, but an increase in incidence of morbidity in HIV-infected children compared with controls has not been shown. Serious bacterial infections due to pyogenic bacteria occur frequently in children with HIV infection (41).

The CDC evaluated the potential effect of requiring serological testing of children before measles immunization and exclusion of HIV-infected children on a hypothetical cohort of one million children in a developing country. It was estimated that this policy would prevent three deaths associated with measles vaccine in HIV-infected children. However, if only 50% of uninfected children return for their immunization, an additional 205 000 cases with 5000 measles deaths would occur (48).

Table 8.4 shows the recommendations for routine immunization of asymptomatic and symptomatic HIV-infected children by the WHO and the Advisory Committee on Immunization Practices (ACIP) of the US Public Health Service. For all children, WHO and ACIP recommend the use of DTP and IPV; ACIP advises against the use of OPV in symptomatic patients. Initially ACIP recommended also that MMR and measles

Table 8.4. *Recommendations on immunization of children infected with human immunodeficiency virus*

Clinical Status	Vaccine				
	BCG	DTP	OPV	IPV	MMR
Symptomatic		*†	*	*†	*†
Asymptomatic	*	*†	*	*†	*†

*Recommended by the World Health Organization.
†Recommended by the Advisory Committee on Immunization Practices of the US Public Health Service.

BCG, bacille Calmette-Guérin vaccine; DTP, diphtheria and tetanus toxoids and pertussis vaccine; OPV, live oral poliovirus vaccine; IPV, inactivated poliovirus vaccine; MMR, measles, mumps and rubella virus vaccine.

vaccine should not be used in symptomatic patients; due to fatal cases of measles reported in unimmunized children and to the absence of adverse reactions, this policy has recently been changed.

In Italy, where BCG is not part of the routine immunization schedule, we do not recommend the use of OPV in infected children, regardless of their clinical status. Moreover, 80–85% of HIV-infected children live with their natural infected parents (9). As family members may be immunocompromised and therefore at increased risk of polio-vaccine-associated paralysis, IPV should be used. Measles vaccine is used in all infected children; hepatitis B vaccine, together with immunoprophylaxis at birth, is recommended for all children born to IVDU mothers, regardless of their serological status.

Diagnosis of infection

Several studies have shown that around 30% of the infants born to HIV-positive women acquire the virus *in utero* or perinatally (10, 17). However, the diagnosis of HIV infection is often difficult. Detection of specific antibodies to the virus is a sensitive and specific indicator of infection in adults, whereas in children the presence of passively transferred antibodies, which have been reported to persist for up to 18 months, limits the diagnostic significance of serology.

In addition to the diagnostic difficulty presented by the persistence of transplacentally derived maternal antibodies, it is often difficult to assess whether the infection has been acquired by infants, or whether symptoms are due to other non-HIV immune problems; for example, congenital B- and T-cell deficiencies must be excluded (7). Moreover, infants born to IVDU mothers frequently show failure to thrive, oral thrush and recurrent infections of the upper respiratory tract without being infected by HIV (49). These infants have lymphocyte abnormalities, suggesting a direct toxic effect of the drug on fetal immunological development (50). On the other hand, CD4/CD8 ratio and total and relative (CD4) lymphocyte counts are not sensitive markers in HIV-infected children (51).

Identification of the virus in the blood or tissues by culture is the method of choice. However, current tests for detection of the virus or its antigens, including cultures, are not standardized and their sensitivity is less than 100%. Thus the CDC has suggested two definitions for paediatric HIV infection (Table 8.5): one for infants and children up to 15 months of age; and another for older children for whom positive serology is

Table 8.5. *Centers for Disease Control (CDC) definition of human immunodeficiency virus (HIV) infection in children less than 13 years of age*

1. Children <15 months of age with perinatal infection have *one* of the following:
   a. HIV in blood or tissues confirmed by culture or other laboratory detection method
   b. Symptoms meeting CDC case definition for acquired immunodeficiency syndrome (AIDS)
   c. Antibody to HIV (repeatedly reactive screening test plus positive confirmatory test result) *and* evidence of both cellular and humoral immunodeficiency (raised immunoglobulin levels, low absolute helper T-cell count, low absolute lymphopenia, low CD4/CD8 ratio) *and* symptoms (class P2)
2. Older perinatally infected children or children who acquired infection through another mode of transmission have *one* of the following:
   a. HIV in blood or tissues confirmed by culture or other laboratory detection method
   b. Antibody to HIV (repeatedly reactive screening test plus positive confirmatory test result)
   c. Symptoms meeting CDC case definition for AIDS

Reproduced from Centers for Disease Control (16).

diagnostic (16). Both definitions use a broad approach based on a global evaluation of children. According to this system, children can be classified as infected, presumably not infected and indeterminate (< 15 months of age, seropositive without clinical and virological evidence of infection).

All children born to HIV-infected mothers are IgG positive at birth. However, only 20–30% of them remain seropositive after 15–18 months of age, suggesting an endogenous production of specific antibodies (10).

Fig. 8.1 shows the loss of specific antibody in 85 children followed from birth in Padua. The mean age at first negative antibody test was 11.3 months (range 3–18 months). Even if all children had a falling antibody titre by 15 months, these data suggest that maternal antibodies can persist up to 18 months of age. Furthermore, in two asymptomatic children who became seronegative at 17 and 18 months, we were able to detect virus reverse transcriptase activity in peripheral blood lymphocyte cultures or the viral genome. This observation, also reported by others, seems to suggest that negative results for HIV IgG do not rule out the diagnosis of infection even in asymptomatic and immunocompetent children at high risk.

The possibility that infants who become seronegative might seroconvert again, has been raised by three reported cases where antibodies appeared after 20 months of age (52). This observation emphasizes the importance of continuous follow-up of all children born to seropositive mothers, regardless of their antibody status.

Detection of specific IgM, an assay used for the diagnosis of other congenital infections, does not seem to be suitable for HIV (53, 54). A prospective study in Zaire of children born to seropositive mothers has shown no correlation between the presence of specific IgM in cord blood and at 3 months of age and the clinical diagnosis of infection (M. Rogers, personal communication).

The *in-vitro* production of specific IgG antibodies (IVAP) against HIV components, described in adults (55), suggests *in-vivo* activation of circulating HIV-specific B cells. This approach has been proposed for children, to detect whether antibodies have been synthesized by the child's lymphocytes or whether they have been passively transferred (56). *In-vitro* IgG antibody production showed a very good predictive value when compared with serology in children over 15 months of age. Similar results have been obtained when IVAP was compared to viral culture.

Recently, a new technique, polymerase chain reaction (PCR), which detects the presence of viral genome integrated in cell DNA through an amplification system, has been proposed for early diagnosis of paediatric HIV infection (57, 58). It presents some

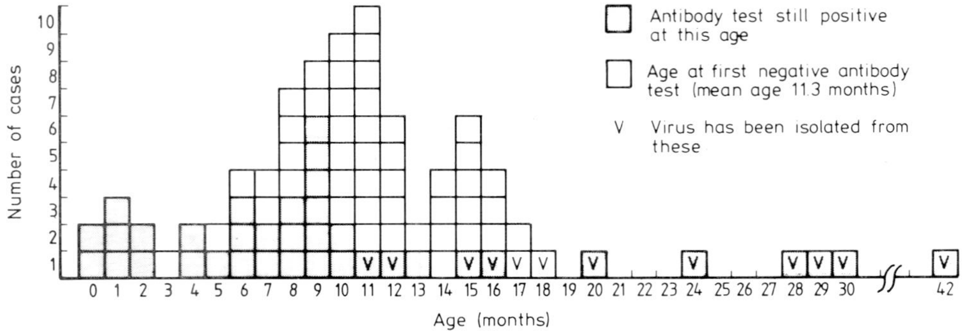

Fig. 8.1. Loss of specific antibody. Results from 85 children followed from birth.

advantages over viral culture, being quicker, less expensive and, above all, very sensitive. Drawbacks are the high risk of contamination and the possibility that some viral strains could escape.

In blood obtained during the neonatal period the PCR was positive in five out of seven infants who later developed AIDS (mean 9.8 months after the test). No proviral sequences were detected in neonatal samples from nine infants who remained well (mean follow-up 16 months) (59). The authors conclude that PCR could be a useful technique to diagnose HIV infection in the newborn, although larger studies are required.

In a series of 101 children born to seropositive mothers we compared IVAP, PCR, viral culture assay and antigenaemia (60). Sixty-four children were repeatedly negative for all parameters, 18 constantly positive and 19 had discordant results. Analysis of the last group revealed the limits of the single diagnostic procedures and also reflected the variable status of HIV infection.

Due to its high sensitivity PCR seems to be very promising for an early diagnosis of HIV infection in infants. However, it must be remembered that even with this test there are false-positive and false-negative results and further studies are needed for improved standardization.

Different antigen-detection techniques have recently been described (61). Although a high sensitivity for antigen capture has been reported, this test reflects an active viral replication which is not always present during the infection (62). Other assays such as *in-situ* hybridization (63), detection of HIV-specific IgG subclasses (64), evaluation of maternal and neonatal Western-blot patterns (65) and detection of secreting antibodies to HIV in neonates (66) have been suggested as diagnostic tools in paediatric infection, but all these techniques need to be further evaluated to determine their sensitivity and specificity for early diagnosis.

The possibility of treating infected newborns with antiviral drugs has been recently raised,

Table 8.6. *Diagnostic evaluation of children born to human immunodeficiency virus (HIV) seropositive mothers*

(a) <*18 months*

HIV-1, HIV-2, HTLV-1 serology	3 monthly
In-vitro antibody production*†	6 monthly
P24 antigenaemia*†	3 monthly
Polymerase chain reaction (PCR)*	6 monthly
Virus culture*	6 monthly

*One confirmed positive test or two positive tests are diagnostic of infection.
†After 2 months of life.

HTLV, human T-lymphotropic virus.

(b) >*18 months*

HIV serology → positive → INFECTED

HIV serology → negative → Antigenaemia, PCR, Virus culture → One confirmed positive or two positive ↓ INFECTED

Antigenaemia, PCR, Virus culture ↓ All negative ↓ NOT INFECTED but to date there is no test which is specific and sensitive enough for an early diagnosis and therefore a broad serological and virological evaluation is essential. Table. 8.6 explains our laboratory approach. However, an overall evaluation of clinical, immunological and laboratory parameters is necessary for the diagnosis of HIV infection in children.

References

1. Centers for Disease Control. Unexplained immunodeficiency and opportunistic infections in infants New York, NJ, California. Morbid Mortal Wkly Rept 1982; 31: 665–7.
2. Centers for Disease Control. AIDS and HIV in the United States: 1988 update. Morbid Mortal Wkly Rep 1989; 38(S4): 1–33.
3. De Rossi A, Della Gassa O, Del Mistro A, Faulkner-Valle GP, Chieco-Bianchi L. HTLV-III and HTLV-I infection in population at risk in the Veneto region of Italy. Eur J Cancer Clin Oncol 1986; 22: 411–18.
4. Mok JQ, Giaquinto C, De Rossi A, Grosch-Worner I, Ades AE, Peckham CS. Infants born to mothers seropositive for human immunodeficiency virus. Lancet 1987; 1: 1164–8.
5. Chiodo F, Ricchi E, Costigliola P, Michelaccoi L, Bovicelli L, Dellacasa P. Vertical transmission of HTLV-III. Lancet 1986; 1: 739.
6. Ziegler JB, Johnson RO, Cooper DA, Gold J. Postnatal transmission of AIDS associated retrovirus from mother to infant. Lancet 1985; 1: 896–7.
7. Falloon J, Edy J, Wiener L, Pizzo P. Human immunodeficiency infection in children. J Pediatr 1989; 114: 1–30.
8. Istituto Superiore di Sanità. AIDS in Italia. Boll Epidemiol Nat 1987; 9: 1–5.
9. Giaquinto C, De Rossi A, D'Elia R et al. Preliminary results of a prospective study on perinatal HIV infection. Riv Inf Ped 1987; 2: 43–9.
10. European Collaborative Study. Mother-to-child transmission of HIV infection. Lancet 1988, 2: 1039–42.
11 Boffey PM. Reagan urges wide AIDS testing but does not call for compulsion. New York Times, 1 June 1987: A1.
12. De Rossi A, Giaquinto C, Zacchello F, Chieco-Bianchi L. Is HIV testing of unselected pregnant women of high priority in Italy? In: Proceedings of the IVth International Conference on AIDS, Stockholm, June 1988. Abstract no. 4633.
13. Meyer KB, Pauker SG. Screening for HIV: can we afford the false positive rate? N Engl J Med 1987; 317: 238–42.
14. Selwyn PA, Schoenbaum EE, Davenny K et al. Prospective study of HIV infection and pregnancy outcomes in intravenous drug abusers. J Am Med Assoc 1989; 261: 1289–94.
15. Vogt MW, Witt DJ, Craven DE, Byngton R, Crawford DF, Schooley RT, Hirsch MS. Isolation of HTLV-III/LAV from cervical secretion of women at risk for AIDS. Lancet 1986; 1: 525–7.
16. Centers for Disease Control. Classification system for human immunodeficiency virus (HIV) infection in children under 13 years of age. Morbid Mortal Wkly Rept 1987; 225–35.
17 Blanche S, Rouzioux C, Guihard-Moscato ML et al. A prospective study of infants born to women seropositive for HIV-1. N Engl J Med 1989; 320: 1643–8.
18. Thiry L, Sprecher-Goldberger S, Jonckheer T et al. Isolation of AIDS virus from cell-free breast milk of three healthy virus carriers. Lancet 1985; 2: 891–2.
19. Centers for Disease Control. Recommendations for assisting in the prevention of perinatal transmission of human immunodeficiency virus and acquired immunodeficiency syndrome. Morbid Mortal Wkly Rep 1985; 34: 721–3.
20. Colebunders RL, Kapita B, Nekwei W et al. Breast feeding and transmission of HIV. In: Proceedings of the IVth International Conference on AIDS, Stockholm, June 1988. Abstract no. 5103.
21. Senturia YD, Ades AE, Peckham CS, Giaquinto C. Breast feeding and HIV infection. Lancet 1987; 2: 400–1.
22. Manzila T, Baende E, Kabagabo U et al. Inability to demonstrate a dose–response effect between receipt of mother's milk and perinatally acquired infection in a cohort of 114 infants born to HIV+ mothers. In: Proceedings of the Vth International Conference on AIDS, Montreal, June 1989, WGO1.
23. Lucas A. Availability of preterm milk. Lancet 1983; 1: 1045–6.

24. Lucas A, Cole TJ, Gore SM *et al.* Multicentre clinical trial of diets for low-birthweight infants: interim analysis of short-term clinical and biochemical effects of diet. Paediatr Res 1984; 18: 807.
25. Lucas A. AIDS and human milk bank closures. Lancet 1987; 1: 1092–3.
26. Eglin RP, Wilkinson AR. HIV infection and pasteurisation of breast milk. Lancet 1987; 1: 1093.
27. Tedder R. HIV infection, breast feeding and human milk banking. Lancet 1988; 2: 452.
28 La Force FM. Immunization of children infected with human immunodeficiency virus: expanded programme on immunization (HIV). Geneva: World Health Organization, 1986: WHO/EPI/86/6.
29. Centers for Disease Control. Immunization of children infected with human T-lymphotropic virus type II/lymphadenopathy associated virus. Morbid Mortal Wkly Rept 1986; 35: 595–605.
30. Onorato IM, Markowitz LE, Oxtoby MJ. Childhood immunization, vaccine preventable diseases and infection with HIV. Pediatr Infect Dis 1988; 7: 588–95.
31. Redfield RR, Wright DC, James WD, Jones TS, Brown C, Burke DS. Disseminated vaccinia in a military recruit with human immunodeficiency virus disease (HIV). N Engl J Med 1987; 316: 673–6.
32. Advisory Committee on Immunization Practices. General recommendations on immunization. Morbid Mortal Wkly Rept 1983; 32: 1–8, 13–17.
33. Halsey NA, Henderson DA. HIV infection against other agents. N Engl J Med 1987; 316: 683–5.
34. Margolick JB, Volkman DDJ, Folks TM et al. Amplification of HTLV-III/LAV infection by antigen induced activation of T cells and direct suppression by virus of lymphocyte blastogenic responses. J Immunol 1987; 138: 1719–23.
35. Buchbinder SP, Hessol N, Lifson A, et al. The interaction of HIV and hepatitis B vaccination in a cohort of homosexual and bisexual men. In: Proceedings of the Vth International Conference on AIDS, Montreal, June 1989. MBP224.
36. Gutfreund K, Chetham-Speth D, Rossol S et al. The effect of vaccination against hepatitis B on the CD4+ cell count in anti-HIV positive men. In: Proceedings of the Vth International Conference on AIDS, Montreal, June 1989. ThBP119.
37. Mvula M, Ryder R, Oxtoby M et al. Measles and measles immunization in African children with HIV. In: Proceedings of the IVth International Conference on AIDS, Stockholm, June 1988. Abstract no. 5112.
38. Mvula M, Ryder R, Manzila T, Matela B. Response to childhood vaccinations in African children with HIV infection. In: Proceedings of the IVth International Conference on AIDS, Stockholm, June 1988. Abstract no. 5107.
39. Blanche S, Le Deist F, Fischer MD et al. Longitudinal study of 18 children with perinatal HTLVIII/LAV infection: attempt at prognostic evaluation. J Pediatr 1986; 109: 965–70.
40. Embrec J, Datta P, Braddick M et al. Vaccination of infants of HIV seropositive mothers. In: Proceedings of the IVth International Conference on AIDS, Stockholm, June 1988. Abstract no. 5108.
41. Bernstein LJ. Ochs HD, Wedgwood RJ et al. Defective humoral immunity in pediatric AIDS. J Pediatr 1985; 107: 352–7.
42. von Reyn CF, Clements CJ, Mann J. HIV infection and routine childhood immunization. Lancet 1987; 2: 689–92.
43. Krasinski K, Borkowsky W, Krugman S. Antibody following measles immunization in children infected with HTLV-III/LAV. In: Proceedings of the IInd International Conference on AIDS, Paris, 23–25 June 1986; 49.
44. Krasinski K, Borkowsky W. Response to polio vaccination in children infected with human immunodeficiency virus. Pediatr Res Soc: 925.
45. Borkowsky W, Steele CJ, Grubman S, Moore T, LaRussa P, Krasinski K. Antibody responses to bacterial toxoids in children infected with human immunodeficiency virus. J Pediatr 1987; 110: 536–6.
46. Mendez H, Fikrig S, DeForest A et al. Response to childhood immunizations in children with HIV infection. In: Proceedings of the IVth International Conference on AIDS, Stockholm, June 1988. Abstract no. 5109.
47. Anderson VM, Kauffman SL, Sher JH et al. The pathology of pediatric AIDS: a review of 33 cases. In: Proceedings of the IIIrd International Conference on AIDS, Washington, June 1987: 138.
48. Onorato IM, Jones TS, Orenstein WA. Immunising children infected with HIV. Lancet 1988; 1: 345–5.
49. Jaffe HW, Feorino PM, Darrow WW et al. Persistent infection with human T-lymphotropic virus type-III lymphadenopathy associated virus

in apparently healthy homosexual men. Ann Intern Med 1985; 102: 627–8.

50. Rosen TS, Johnson HL. Children with methadone-maintained mothers: follow up to 18 months of age. J Pediatr 1982; 101: 192–6.
51. Culver KW, Ammann AJ, Colin Partridge J, Wong DF, Wara DW, Cowan MJ. Lymphocyte abnormalities in infants born to drug abusing mothers. J Pediatr 1987; 111: 230–5.
52. Aiuti F, Luzi G, Mezzaroma I, Scano G, Papetti C. Delayed appearance of HIV infection in children.
53 Landesman S, Mendez H, Bigger B et al. Evaluation of HIV IgM and antigen assays for determination of perinatal infection with HIV. In: Proceedings of the IIIrd International Conference on AIDS, Washington, 1–5 June 1987. THP71.
54. Gaetano C, Scano G, Carbonari M et al. Delayed and defective anti-HIV IgM response in infants. Lancet 1987; 1: 631.
55. Amadori A, De Rossi A, Faulkner Valle G et al. Spontaneous *in vitro* production of virus specific antibody by lymphocytes from HIV infected subjects. Clin Immunol Immunopathol 1988; 46: 342–51.
56. Amadori A, De Rossi A, Giaquinto C et al. *In vitro* production of HIV infected antibody in children at risk of AIDS. Lancet 1988; 1: 852–4.
57. De Rossi A, Amadori A, Chieco-Bianchi L et al. Polymerase chain reaction and 'in vitro' antibody production for early diagnosis of pediatric HIV infection. Lancet 1988; 2: 278.
58. Laure F, Courgnaud V, Rouzioux C et al. Detection of HIV1 DNA in infants and children by means of the polymerase chain reaction. Lancet 1988; 2: 538–41.
59. Rogers M, Chin-Yih O, Rayfield M et al. Use of the polymerase chain reaction for early detection of the proviral sequences of HIV in infants born to seropositive mothers. N Engl J Med 1989; 320: 1649–54.
60. De Rossi A, Giaquinto C, Amadori A et al. Early diagnosis of HIV infection in children born to seropositive mothers. International Conference on AIDS, Montreal, June 1989. TBP244.
61. Borkowsky W, Krasinski K, Paul D et al. Human immunodeficiency virus infections in infants negative for anti HIV by enzyme-linked immunoassay. Lancet 1987; 1: 1168–70.
62. Haseltine WA. Silent HIV infections. N Engl J Med 1989; 320: 1487–9.
63. Harnish DG, Hamerberg O, Walker IR et al. Early detection of HIV infection in newborn. N Engl J Med 1987; 316: 273.
64. Pyun KH, Ochs HD, Dufford MTW, Wedgwood RJ. Perinatal infection with human immunodeficiency virus: specific antibody responses by the neonate. N Engl J Med 1987; 317: 611–13.
65. Mendez H, Holman S, Stevens R et al. ELISA and Western blot patterns and a possible marker of seroreversion in infants born to seropositive women. In: Proceedings of the Vth International Conference on AIDS, Montreal, June 1989. TBP240.
66. Archibald D, Nair P, Hines S, Davis E, Johnson J. Detection of secretory antibodies to HIV in neonates. In: Proceedings of the Vth International Conference on AIDS, Montreal, June 1989. TBP238.

9 Septicaemia and Meningitis in the Newborn

J. de Louvois
Queen Charlotte's and Chelsea Hospital, London, UK

Neonatal sepsis is reported to affect up to 1% of babies, half of whom may be expected to have septicaemia (1), and it is suggested that one in five septicaemic babies develop meningitis. These figures can be no more than a general indication of the extent of neonatal sepsis, which varies considerably from place to place. Reports on the results of bacterial cultures collected *post mortem* indicate that in some centres a significant proportion of neonatal sepsis goes unrecognized and is only revealed at autopsy (2, 3). The size of this problem is unknown since postmortem examination of babies who die is not a routine investigation in many hospitals. Even when autopsies are performed, cultures of heart blood, cerebro-spinal fluid (CSF) and bronchus are not always examined.

Neonatal septicaemia is more common in preterm and low-birthweight babies; in many neonatal intensive care units (NICUs) the incidence may be as high as 10%, with a correspondingly high incidence of cases of meningitis. The practice of concentrating low-birthweight and preterm babies in specialist units and of transferring them *in utero* rather than after birth may give a falsely low impression of the level of neonatal sepsis in non-specialist centres and depressingly high levels of sepsis in specialist centres.

A newborn baby, especially if born prematurely, is highly susceptible to infection and, because the immune systems are underdeveloped, may be prey to many bacteria that in older patients would not be pathogenic. The range and distribution of bacteria isolated from neonatal blood are constantly changing and will vary from nursery to nursery. It is therefore essential that each unit should maintain detailed information on the frequency, type and antibiotic sensitivity of bacteria isolated from the newborn. Blood-culture isolates from babies admitted to the NICU at Queen Charlotte's and Chelsea Hospital in recent years are shown in Table 9.1. The most notable feature is the increasing incidence of infection due to *Staphylococcus epidermidis* and similar coagulase-negative gram-positive cocci. It is clear that, within our unit, infection with the Lancefield group B streptococcus (GBS; *Streptococcus agalactiae*), enterococci and *Listeria monocytogenes* has not constituted a major problem. Environmental bacteria, such as *Pseudomonas aeruginosa*, *Enterobacter* spp. and *Serratia* spp., although isolated from time to time, have not been responsible for major outbreaks of infection.

The aseptic collection of blood from small babies is not easy and is further complicated by the fact that *Staph. epidermidis*, now the commonest cause of neonatal septicaemia in many units, is also a common commensal on the hands of staff. Thus without scrupulous care the blood sample may be contaminated

Infection in the Newborn. Edited by J. de Louvois and D. Harvey
©1990 John Wiley & Sons Ltd

Table 9.1. *Positive blood cultures (Queen Charlotte's and Chelsea Hospital, 1979–1988)*

	1979	1983	1984	1985	1987	1988
Coagulase-negative staph.	7	4	2	19	14	29
Coagulase-positive staph.	1	1	2	2	1	4
Group B streptococci	1	1	3	3	3	2
Listeria monocytogenes	1	—	—	—	1	3
Enterococci	—	—	3	—	1	1
Escherichia coli	4	3	1	2	2	—
Klebsiella spp.	—	—	—	3	—	—
Enterobacter spp.	1	1	2	1	3	—
Pseudomonas aeruginosa	2	—	1	—	1	—
Serratia spp.	1	1	—	—	1	—
Other	—	4	5	5	2	8
Gram-negative rods	1	—	1	3	1	—
Bacteraemic babies	19	15	20	30	28	32
Admissions to NICU	268	256	228	289	227	326
Bacteraemic babies (%)	7.0	5.8	8.7	10.4	12.3	9.8

NICU, Neonatal Intensive Care Unit.

by the collector. Contamination of a blood culture may also occur from organisms on the baby's skin, especially when cultures are collected shortly after birth. Two separate antiseptic wipes should be used to prepare the puncture site. We have found it useful also to swab the site after the sample of blood has been drawn. Any bacteria isolated from the skin can then be matched with the blood-culture isolate, thus greatly assisting the interpretation of blood-culture results. Whenever possible, blood for culture should be collected by venepuncture. A new needle must be fitted to the syringe before the sample is inoculated into blood-culture bottles. Inoculation must be through the diaphragm of the cap, which must first be disinfected with an alcohol swab. Under no circumstances should the cap of the culture bottle be removed, nor must the blood sample be used for blood-gas analysis before being added to the culture bottles. Outbreaks of 'pseudo-sepsis' have been reported as a result of bacteria from the blood-gas analyser contaminating the blood sample before inoculation into the culture medium. Laboratory contamination, which in the past has also been a problem, can be largely eliminated by removing all subculture samples through the diaphragm by means of syringe and needle. Caution should be exercised regarding the use of the newer non-sampling methods of blood culture, such as the Signal Blood Culture System marketed by Oxoid, since many of the isolates from neonatal blood fail to trigger the indicator system. Blood samples collected by needle stab or via an intravenous line must only be used for bacterial culture under extreme circumstances and positive results from such specimens must be interpreted with great caution.

Cord blood for culture can be collected aseptically at the time of delivery; but this has not been common in the UK. It has the great advantage that a much larger volume of blood is available than can reasonably be collected from the baby. The very limited volume of blood available from small babies is a major problem in the accurate diagnosis of early septicaemia. It is not uncommon for the first sample of blood from babies with clinical signs of septicaemia or shock to be negative, but for bacteria to be isolated from subsequent samples, thus emphasizing the need to collect more than one blood culture from ill neonates.

Because the risk of contamination is high, it is usually only possible to collect a single blood culture before initiating antibiotic therapy and, because many of the isolates associated with bacteraemia are also common saprophytes, criteria must be established for deciding whether or not a blood-culture isolate is significant. In our practice, coagulase-negative staphylococci and similar low-grade pathogens must be isolated in pure culture from both bottles of a blood-culture set, and not from the puncture-site swab, before they are considered to be significant. Subsequently both organisms must be shown to have the same sensitivity pattern. Mixed bacterial populations and anaerobic bacteria are infrequently associated with bacteraemia in the newborn, except possibly in cases of intestinal perforation. These bacteria are, however, commonly found as skin contaminants in early neonatal life and when they are grown from blood samples the possibility of contamination at the time of collection must be considered. It should be remembered also that fastidious microorganisms, such as *Mycoplasma hominis* and *Bacteriodes* spp., which a baby encounters during the birth process, may survive for quite long periods on preterm newborn skin.

Septicaemia

Septicaemia may arise *in utero*, or at any time during the neonatal period. When infection arises *in utero* or during the first 3 days of life, it is most probable that bacteria from the mother's genital tract, notably GBS or *Escherichia coli*, are responsible. After the first few days of life, organisms from the environment, such as *Ps. aeruginosa*, *Serratia* spp. or *Enterobacter* spp., or from the hands of those handling the baby, such as *Staph. epidermidis*, are most likely to be implicated. It is apparent from Table 9.1 that early-onset infection originating from maternal sources is not a major problem in our unit, the bulk of septicaemia rising as an indirect consequence of intensive care.

Knowledge of the microbes most commonly implicated in septicaemia and of their antibiotic sensitivity patterns allows rational decisions to be made regarding the antibiotic regimen to be employed within the NICU for the 'blind' treatment of clinically septic babies. Units in which early neonatal sepsis is common may find it useful to have one antibiotic regimen for babies less than 4 days old and another for older babies. It is general practice in the UK, however, for units to have a single regimen for 'blind' therapy and to modify this, if necessary, when culture results are available. We have been unhappy about the random use of the aminoglycosides in the newborn and, aware of the difficulties of maintaining safe therapeutic serum concentrations of gentamicin in small babies (4), it has been our practice for many years to rely on monotherapy with one of the third-generation cephalosporins for 'blind' antibiotic therapy in the newborn (5–9). The high percentage of hospital isolates of gram-negative rods which are resistant to ampicillin and the increasing resistance to gentamicin among the coagulase-negative staphylococci give rise to concern about the use of an ampicillin/gentamicin combination for 'blind' therapy in centres which do not have major problems with infection due to GBS or listeria. In our NICU, bacterial isolates from cases of septicaemia are more often sensitive to cefotaxime than to the ampicillin/gentamicin combination. The third-generation cephalosporins have the advantage also of not needing to be monitored and of achieving therapeutic concentrations in CSF even when the meninges are not inflamed, at least in early neonatal life (10). During the 3-year period 1983–1985, in which cephalosporins were being used routinely for initial therapy in the NICU, no case of meningitis occurred in 773 babies, 8% of whom weighed less than 1000 g at birth. During this time 74/773 (9.6%) babies on the unit had bacteraemia.

The mortality associated with septicaemia ranges from 10 to 70%, depending on the age and degree of prematurity of the baby. The higher mortality rates are associated with intrauterine and early neonatal sepsis, especially when due to GBS and in cases that progress to meningitis. Despite new antibiotics and improvements in intensive care, neurodevelopmental impairment is seen in up to 20% of survivors of septicaemia and even more often after meningitis. This is due in part to the difficulty of early diagnosis and in part to the impaired immunological competence of the newborn. This is manifest in reduced plasma opsonic activity (11), defects in the number and function of granulocytes (12) and deficient cell-mediated immunity (13). The transfusion of whole blood or plasma has been used to good effect in the treatment of septicaemia (14). It is not clear whether the beneficial effect of simple or exchange transfusion lies in providing added opsonic activity and antibody against the infecting micro-organism or is due to the effects of increasing the blood volume, blood pressure and tissue perfusion and the better oxygen transport provided by adult haemoglobin. In neonatal sepsis the marrow stores of neutrophils are rapidly mobilized, but they are only replenished slowly. Thus exhaustion of the marrow with resultant neutropenia is a common consequence of serious infection in the newborn. It is therefore attractive to consider transfusing mature granulocytes to babies with septicaemia (15).

A number of controlled studies now attest to the value of granulocyte transfusion in the treatment of septicaemia (15–17). All of these studies report significantly lower mortality in babies who received granulocyte transfusions and an absence of graft-versus-host reactions or other side-effects.

Attempts have been made to prevent sepsis in preterm and low-birthweight babies by administering immunoglobulin at the time of delivery (18). In a controlled study a significantly lower sepsis rate was reported in babies who received 120 mg/kg immunoglobulin intravenously at birth or on days 1 and 8 of life compared to controls matched for birthweight. No adverse effects of serotherapy were noted during the study or at follow-up at the age of 6 months. An alternative approach to improving the host defences of the neonate has been to consider vaccinating mothers known to be antibody deficient against GBS. A vaccine prepared from the capsular polysaccharide of type III GBS is immunogenic in man (19). Thus active immunization during pregnancy, of mothers known to be antibody deficient against this organism, might be expected to boost antibody levels of both mother and baby and reduce the probability of GBS sepsis. The value of this approach must be considered by individual units according to the incidence of early-onset streptococcal infection.

Meningitis

Opinions are divided about the need for routine lumbar punctures (LPs) on all babies considered to be septic. Pearse and Roberton (20) assert that an LP 'should be performed in all babies where there is a possibility of meningitis'. They go on to propose that 'since it is impossible to rule out meningitis clinically and because babies with suspected sepsis should not be started on antibiotics without knowing whether the CSF is infected, a lumbar puncture is nearly always performed'. Concern has been expressed about the practice of a routine LP in all babies showing signs of sepsis, and Harper (21) and McWilliam (22) caution against the procedure in babies or children with raised intracranial pressure or decreased levels of consciousness. There is a body of opinion also that asserts that, if the results of a CSF examination are not going

Table 9.2. *Meningitis among 62 107 newborn infants (London and Bristol, 1979–1985)*

	Weight at birth (kg)					
	<1.0		1.0–1.5		>1.5	
Total number of babies	263		510		61 334	
Babies who had lumbar puncture	122	(46%)	216	(42%)	746	(1%)
Number of lumbar punctures	276		364		914	
Babies with meningitis (total)	3		2		12	
Meningitis in first 3 days of life	2*		1*		5	
Incidence per 100 live births	11.0		3.9		0.2	
Mortality from meningitis (%)	66		50		0	
CSF samples positive (%)	1.6		1.5		1.5	

*3/57 (5.3%) who had lumbar punctures in the first 3 days of life.

CSF, cerebrospinal fluid.

to alter clinical management of the individual neonate, then an LP should not be performed. The possible benefits of routine LPs have not been determined, although a number of risk factors have been identified. An LP may initiate meningitis in babies who are bacteraemic (23), induce coning in patients with raised intracranial pressure (24) and, in very small babies, result in damage to the spinal cord (J. Pryse-Davies, unpublished). If a needle without a stylet is used, there is a risk that an intraspinal epidermoid tumour may develop later in life (25). Even in the absence of these major complications, LP of a sick neonate may bring about a reduction in blood-gas tensions (26) or major clinical deterioration (27).

A recent study (28) has examined the value of LPs carried out in three major neonatal centres over a period of 6 years (Table 9.2). Each centre had a restrictive policy with regard to the collection of CSF from premature babies. Lumbar puncture was only performed when there was clinical evidence suggestive of meningitis and it did not form part of the routine investigation upon admission. Thus, among 773 babies weighing less than 1500 g at birth, only 57 (7.4%) had an LP during the first 3 days of life and more than 50% of such babies did not have an LP at any time during their stay in the NICU. Meningitis was diagnosed in 17 of 1084 babies who had an LP; only five of these 17 were in the very low birthweight (VLBW) group under 1500 g. It can be argued that there were other babies with meningitis who, not having had an LP, were treated adequately by the routine antibiotic regimen for the treatment of sepsis in the newborn. There was no evidence that undiagnosed cases of meningitis were being found at autopsy, as has been reported from other centres (2, 3). In one of the centres involved in the study by MacMahon et al. (28), 90% of babies who died during the study period came to autopsy, and samples of CSF, heart blood and a bronchial swab were collected as part of the autopsy routine. There was no evidence from these cultures that meningitis or septicaemia was being missed in life. In this study the three VLBW babies with positive CSF cultures had CSF white-cell counts of less than 3 cells/μl, a finding confirmed recently by other workers (29).

The incidence of meningitis in the newborn in Great Britain has until recently been unknown. Figures from the Office of Population Censuses and Surveys and from the Communicable Diseases Surveillance Centre give an underestimate of the true incidence. Even in cases of meningococcal meningitis, which is statutorily notifiable, there is considerable under-reporting. We have recently completed a 2-year national survey of meningitis in children under 1 year of age.

Table 9.3. *Neonatal meningitis (Great Britain, 1985–1987)*

	Number of cases where isolated
N. meningitis	14
H. influenzae	12
Strep. pneumoniae	21
Strep. agalactiae (GBS)	113
E. coli	82
L. monocytogenes	21
Proteus spp.	8
Enterobacter spp.	3
Salmonella spp.	2
Klebsiella spp.	5
Serratia spp.	4
Citrobacter spp.	4
Acinetobacter spp.	1
Pseudomonas spp.	3
'Coliforms'	5
Staph. aureus	4
Staph. epidermidis	9
Faecal streptococci	6
β-haemolytic streptococci (other)	2
Other bacteria	11
Echoviruses	7
Other viruses	5
Sterile CSF	125
CSF not taken	9

GBS, group B streptococci; CSF, cerebrospinal fluid.

The results suggest that there are between 150 and 200 cases of meningitis per year in babies under 28 days of age (0.4/1000 live births), significantly above the figure of 100 cases per year which is widely quoted for the UK. The bacterial isolates most frequently encountered in this study are shown in Table 9.3. It can be seen that GBS is significantly more common than *E. coli*, thus confirming the increasing importance in recent years of GBS as a cause of neonatal meningitis in Great Britain. Of interest also are the relatively large number of cases of neonatal meningitis which were due to *Neisseria meningitidis*, *Haemophilus influenzae* and *Streptococcus pneumoniae*, the bacterial species most commonly responsible for meningitis in older children, and the finding that many of these occurred during the first 48 h of life. These organisms accounted for 13% of the total number of cases. Although meningitis of viral origin is not uncommon in the newborn, large numbers of laboratories do not include virus culture among their routine investigations, even when these facilities are available. Many of the clinical cases of meningitis in which the cultures were negative may have been uninvestigated viral infections.

Although 33% of culture-positive cases were due to GBS, they only accounted for 22% of deaths, whereas *E. coli*, with 22% cases, accounted for 25% of deaths. In total, 106 cases were due to enteric gram-negative rods and 32 (30%) patients died. This confirms previous reports that meningitis due to enteric gram-negative rods has a higher mortality than that due to gram-positive organisms. There was only one death among the 21 cases of meningitis due to *L. monocytogenes.*

In this study the overall mortality in cases of culture-positive meningitis was 23%, which is comparable to the figure from our previous prospective study (30). The mortality rate among the culture-negative cases is also comparable: 3% in this study compared to 5% previously. None of the 12 cases of viral meningitis died. Thus in the absence of viable bacteria in the CSF the prognosis is good. Many of the babies whose CSF was sterile had received antibiotics from the referring physician prior to admission to hospital. The low mortality rate among these babies emphasizes the importance of early treatment in the successful management of meningitis in the newborn period.

The morbidity associated with meningitis has yet to be determined for the national study; however, in our previous study (30) it exceeded 20% for both the culture-positive and the culture-negative group of patients. The finding of significant neurological deficit in more than 20% of survivors is in agreement with the results of other prospective studies in the newborn (31).

The rapid diagnosis of meningitis in the newborn remains a problem. There are commercial reagents which rapidly detect antigenic components of the bacteria most frequently associated with meningitis in older children: *Strep. pneumoniae*, *H. influenzae* and *N. meningitidis*. With the exception of GBS, similar reagents are not available for the rapid diagnosis of meningitis in the newborn.

The reagents currently available are based on slide agglutination of antibody-coated particles (latex or staphylococci). They are designed to give early recognition of bacteria, which can subsequently be cultured. Given the very high activity that can be achieved with monoclonal antibodies, it is unfortunate that manufacturers have not shown more interest in producing reagents that are as sensitive as possible, within the limits of specificity, rather than directing their energies only towards samples that contain sufficient bacteria to give a positive culture result. The wide range of bacteria responsible for meningitis in the newborn and the relatively low number of cases per year in Western Europe make it unlikely that specific reagents will be produced. However, it ought to be possible to produce high-activity monoclonal antibodies against gram-negative lipopolysaccharide and thus provide the means of recognizing infection due to gram-negative enteric rods.

In the UK, chloramphenicol is still the antibiotic most widely used for the treatment of meningitis. Recent studies have highlighted the problems of inappropriate dosage, incorrect administration and inadequate monitoring of serum concentrations (32, 33). Seventeen (7.8%) of patients in the latter study were known to have received an overdose and in others the prescription differed significantly from that recommended. Six neonates developed the 'grey baby syndrome' and three of these died. Six older children developed haematological changes; none died. Five babies who received 2–10 times the prescribed dosage of chloramphenicol suffered no discernible ill effects. Transient serum concentrations above the therapeutic range of 15–25 mg/l are not associated with toxicity; problems arise when high concentrations are maintained for long periods. Even in small babies who receive the correct parenteral dose the resultant serum concentration is totally unpredictable. Among such babies 25% will have serum concentrations above the therapeutic range and in 50% the serum concentrations will be subtherapeutic (32). In small babies the situation is further complicated by variation in the rate at which chloramphenicol succinate is de-esterified following intravenous injection. High-performance liquid chromatographic assay methods for chloramphenicol can easily be modified to measure both chloramphenicol and chloramphenicol succinate, and thus avoid misinterpretation of assay results because of unrecognized succinate. In our 2-year prospective national study 48% of the neonates had antibiotic regimens based on chloramphenicol; in 24% the regimen was based on gentamicin and in 14% on cefotaxime. Many babies received combinations of two or more of these agents. A total of 106 out of 409 (26%) neonates received antibiotic combinations which included cefotaxime or ceftazidime. This is in contrast to our previous study in which all the babies received chloramphenicol with or without gentamicin or ampicillin. This difference probably reflects a move away from chloramphenicol therapy in referral hospitals and the satisfactory results reported after the use of third generation cephalosporins in the treatment of paediatric meningitis (34–38). The anticipated serum and CSF concentrations of some of the newer antimicrobial agents

Table 9.4. *New antibiotics used in the treatment of meningitis—antibacterial activity in cerebrospinal fluid (CSF)*

Antibiotic	Peak serum concentration (mg/l)	CSF/serum ratio (%)	Peak CSF concentration (mg/l)	Predicted CSF bactericidal activity		
				E. coli	GBS	Listeria
Ceftazidime	125	12	15	15–30	15–30	<1
Cefotaxime	100	10	10	20–40	40–80	<1
Moxalactam	125	20	25	50–100	1–2	<1
Ceftriaxone	175	7	12	50–100	25–50	<1
Cefoperazone	125	6	7.5	1	40–80	<1

GBS, group B streptococci.

following a standard dose are shown in Table 9.4. It can be seen that for all of these agents except moxalactam the CSF should contain more than 20 times the concentration required to kill *E. coli* and GBS. None of these agents are clinically active against listeria, for which the treatment of choice remains ampicillin or penicillin and gentamicin.

References

1. Chiswick ML. Infection and de-fences in neonates. Br Med J 1983; 1: 1377–8.
2. Pierce JR, Merenstein GB, Stocker JT. Immediate postmortem cultures in an intensive care nursery. Pediatr Infect Dis 1984; 3: 510–13.
3. Eisenfeld L, Ermocilla R, Wirtschafter D, Cassady G. Systemic bacterial infections in neonatal deaths. Am J Dis Child 1983; 137: 645–9.
4. Mulhall A, de Louvois J, Hurley R. Incidence of potentially toxic concentrations of gentamicin in the neonate. Arch Dis Child 1983; 58: 897–900.
5. de Louvois J, Mulhall A, Hurley R. Cefuroxime in the treatment of neonates. Arch Dis Child 1982; 57: 59–62.
6. de Louvois J, Mulhall A, James J. Latamoxef in the newborn. Arch Dis Child 1984; 59: 346–50.
7. de Louvois J, Mulhall A, Hurley R. The safety and pharmacokinetics of cefotaxime in the treatment of neonates. Pediatr Pharmacol 1982; 2: 275–84.
8. Pollock I, Mulhall A, de Louvois J. Ceftazidime in the treatment of neonatal infection. J Hosp Infect 1985; 6: 158–65.
9. James J, Mulhall A, de Louvois J. Ceftriaxone—clinical experience in the treatment of neonates. J Infect 1985; 11: 25–33.
10. de Louvois J. Serious infection in the newborn. Hospital Update 1985; Serious Infections Series No. 7. Update Group, London.
11. Miller ME. Phagocytosis in the newborn infant: humoral and cellular factors. J Pediatr 1969; 74: 255–9.
12. Christensen RD, Anstall HB, Rothstein G. Review: deficiencies in the neutrophil system of newborn infants, and the use of leukocyte transfusion in the treatment of neonatal sepsis. J Clin Apheresis 1982; 1: 33–41.
13. Chandra RK. Serum thymic hormone activity and cell-mediated immunity in healthy neonates, preterm infants, and small-for-gestational age infants. Pediatrics 1981; 67: 407–11.
14. Vain NE, Mazhumian JR, Swarner W, Cha CC. Role of exchange transfusion in the treatment of severe septicaemia. Pediatrics 1980; 66: 693–7.
15. Chistensen RD, Rothstein G, Anstall HB, Bybee B. Granulocyte transfusions in neonates with bacterial infection, neutropenia, and depletion of mature marrow neutrophils. Pediatrics 1982; 70: 1–6.
16. Laurenti F, Ferro R, Isacchi G et al. Polymorphonuclear leukocyte transfusion for the treatment of sepsis in the newborn infant. J Pediatr 1981; 98: 118–23.
17. Cairo MS, Rucker R, Bennetts GA, Hicks D, Worcester C, Amlie R et al. Improved survival of newborns receiving leucocyte transfusions for sepsis. Pediatrics 1984; 74: 887–92.

18. Haque KN, Zaidi MH, Haque SK et al. Intravenous immunoglobulin for prevention of sepsis in preterm and low birth weight infants. Pediatr Infect Dis 1986; 5: 622–5.
19. Baker CJ, Edwards MS, Kasper DL. Immunogenicity of polysaccharides from type III group B streptococcus. J Clin Invest 1978; 61: 1107–10.
20. Pearse RG, Roberton NRC. Infection in the newborn. In: Roberton NRC (ed). Textbook of neonatology. London: Churchill Livingstone, 1986: 725–81.
21. Harper JR. Timing of lumbar puncture in severe childhood meningitis. Br Med J 1985; 2: 651.
22. McWilliam R. Timing of lumbar puncture in severe childhood meningitis. Br Med J 1985; 2: 1124.
23. Teele DW, Dashefsky B, Rakusan T, Klein JO. Meningitis after lumbar puncture in children with bacteremia. N Engl J Med 1981; 305: 1079–81.
24. Harper JR, Lorber J, Hillas-Smith G, Bower BD, Eykyn SJ. Timing of lumbar puncture in severe childhood meningitis. Br Med J 1985; 291: 651–2.
25. Choremis C, Economos D, Papadatos C, Gargoulas A. Intraspinal tumours (cholesteatomas) in patients treated for tuberculous meningitis. Lancet 1956; 2: 437.
26. Gleason CA, Martin RJ, Anderson JV, Waldermar AC, Sanniti KJ, Fanaroff AA. Optimal position for a spinal tap in preterm infants. Pediatrics 1983; 71: 31–5.
27. Weisman LE, Merenstein GB, Steenbarger JR. The effect of lumbar puncture position in sick neonates. Am J Dis Child 1983; 137: 1077–9.
28. MacMahon P, Jewes L, de Louvois J. Routine lumbar puncture in the newborn – are they justified? Eur J Pediatr (in press).
29. Revell P, Cann K. Clinical justification for cerebrospinal fluid investigation. Lancet 1987; 1: 221.
30. Mulhall A, de Louvois J, Hurley R. Efficacy of chloramphenicol in the treatment of neonatal and infantile meningitis: a study of 70 cases. Lancet 1983; 1: 284–7.
31. Klein JO, Feigin RD, McCracken GH. Report of the task force on diagnosis and management of meningitis. Pediatrics 1986; 78: 959–82.
32. Mulhall A, de Louvois J, Hurley R. The pharmacokinetics of chloramphenicol in the neonate and young infant. J Antimicrob Chemother 1983; 12: 629–39.
33. Mulhall A, de Louvois J, Hurley R. Chloramphenicol toxicity in the neonate: its incidence and prevention. Br Med J 1983; 2: 1424–7.
34. Eichenwald HF. Bacterial meningitis: is there a 'best' antimicrobial therapy? Eur J Pediatr 1987; 146: 216–20.
35. McCracken GH Jr, Threlkeid N, Mize SG et al. Moxalactam therapy for neonatal meningitis due to gram-negative enteric bacilli: a prospective controlled evaluation. J Am Med Assoc 1984; 252: 1427–32.
36. Odio CM, Faingezicht I, Salas JL, Guevara J, Mohs E, McCracken GH Jr. Cefotaxime vs conventional therapy for the treatment of bacterial meningitis of infants and children. Pediatr Infect Dis 1986; 5: 402–7.
37. Rodriguez WJ, Puig JR, Khan WN, Feris J, Gold BG, Sturia C. Ceftazidime vs standard therapy for pediatric meningitis: therapeutic, pharmacologic and epidemiologic observations. Pediatr Infect Dis 1986; 5: 408–15.
38. Modai J, Meulemans A, Vittecoq D. Treatment of *Pseudomonas aeruginosa* meningitis with ceftazidime. J Antimicrob Chemoth 1983; 11: 198–9.

10 Immunoglobulin Therapy in Neonatal Sepsis

K. N. Haque
Division of Neonatology, Department of Paediatrics, College of Medicine, Riyadh, Saudi Arabia

Introduction

The newborn human infant is prone to bacterial infection (1–4). There are a number of reasons for this enhanced susceptibility: antibody deficiency (5–7), low levels of complement for both the classical and the alternate pathway (8–10), reduced fibronectin levels (11, 12), a decreased neutrophil storage pool (13), defective neutrophil function (11, 14), and altered production, release and chemotaxis of polymorphonuclear neutrophils (15, 16).

Despite better perinatal care, early diagnosis and use of broad-spectrum antibiotics, the mortality from neonatal sepsis is still in excess of 30–50% in most reported series (3, 4, 17, 18). Mortality from neonatal sepsis is highest among very low birthweight infants (19, 20). It is for these extremely premature infants, as well as for those infants who appear septic at the time of or soon after birth (and who may rapidly succumb), that additional types of therapy have been sought.

Steen (21) and Amer et al. (22) were the first to use gammaglobulins as therapeutic agents in preterm infants with sepsis. Unfortunately the preparations they used were crude in comparison to what are available today, and their results were equivocal. Recent interest in immunoglobulins as therapeutic agents in neonatal sepsis has evolved primarily through advances in our understanding of the role of type-specific antibody. Although the capacity for antibody synthesis exists early in gestation (IgM, 10 weeks; IgG and IgE, 12 weeks; IgA, 30 weeks), the newborn infant produces very little of his or her own immunoglobulin due to: (1) inadequate processing of antigen by macrophages; (2) lack of antigenic stimulation *in utero*; and (3) increased numbers of suppressor T cells which inhibit antibody synthesis (23). The newborn infant is thus totally dependent on active transport of IgG across the placenta for protective antibodies. Immunoglobulin is mainly transferred to the fetus during the last few weeks before birth (24). Moreover, serum IgG levels begin to fall immediately after birth. Hence infants born prematurely are deprived of protective antibodies, and their specific immune systems (antibody production and T cells) are too slow to have an impact on bacterial disease in the neonatal period (25). In addition to the lack of protective antibodies, Christensen and others (26–30) have shown abnormalities in the cell morphology, changes in the concentration of circulating neutrophils and deficiencies in the neutrophil storage pool, consisting of polymorphonuclear neutrophils, band cells and metamyelocytes, in neonates with bacterial sepsis (13). Given the above deficiencies in the defence mechanisms of the newborn, particularly the preterm, and the deficiencies

Infection in the Newborn. Edited by J. de Louvois and D. Harvey
©1990 John Wiley & Sons Ltd

in the neonate's response to sepsis, it is little wonder that the rate of infection and mortality from neonatal sepsis is high.

Gammaglobulin therapy

Treatment with gammaglobulins is based on the principle of supplementing the antibody reserves of a non-immune recipient, who either is at risk of infection or has an infectious disease with serum antibody from an immunized donor. This process was developed over a 100 years ago by Emil von Behring, who used immune horse serum to treat patients with tetanus and diphtheria. Due to the considerable side-effects and the shortcomings of the method, the use of antibodies from immunized donors did not become an established form of treatment of infectious disease. However, the theoretical arguments for the use of immunoglobulins are very strong (25). Passive intravenous immunoglobulin (IVIg) preparations provide a rapid and effective method for increasing serum immunoglobulin levels in neonates (31). Antibody enhances phagocytosis, inhibits bacterial adhesion, neutralizes toxins and activates complement, which in turn enhances opsonization (32). More recently it has been shown that IVIg accelerates the release of mature neutrophils from the storage pool and marrow reserves (33).

Steen (21) studied two groups of preterm infants to determine the number of infections contracted during the first year of life. The group who had received bimonthly intramuscular gammaglobulin injections had a similar number of infections to the group who did not receive gammaglobulin. Amer et al. (22) followed up 92 infants who had received a monthly intramuscular injection of immune serum globulin and found that they experienced a reduced number of minor infections compared to a placebo-treated group. There was, however, no difference in the number of serious infections and neonatal deaths. The immune serum globulin used in the studies by Steen (21) and Amer et al. (22) was a viscous (16.5 g/dl) solution requiring deep intramuscular injection. This not only was very painful, but also led to severe local reactions. These reactions were probably secondary to aggregated immunoglobulin particles in the preparations – such particles can activate anticomplement activity. Moreover, systemic absorption of intramuscular serum globulin is highly variable and it takes several days for tissue levels to equilibrate following an injection.

The availability of immunoglobulins for intravenous use, and more importantly the availability of preparations with an intact and stable Fc fraction, has eliminated the anticomplementary activity of the previous preparations and has led to renewed interest in the use of immunoglobulins as therapeutic agents. Sidiropolous et al. (34) was the first to report the successful use of IVIg in the treatment of neonatal sepsis. In a study of 35 infected newborn infants they reported a decrease in mortality rate in a group who received IVIg plus antibiotics as compared to a control group who received antibiotics alone (Table 10.1). Although the overall result was not statistically significant, mortality in preterm infants was significantly reduced in the IVIg-treated group (4/9 died in the group receiving antibiotics alone compared with 1/13 in the group receiving antibiotics plus IVIg; *P* 0.04).

Since 1981 various workers (35) have studied the efficacy and pharmacokinetics of IVIg in neonatal sepsis and performed animal protection studies with type III group B streptococci (GBS) (36). The pharmacokinetics of various IVIg preparations and their effects against GBS have been extensively studied (37–39). The long-term effects of IVIg have been studied by Sidiropolous et al. (34) and others, who have found no untoward effects in terms of psychomotor development,

Table 10.1. *Results of intravenous immunoglobulin (IVIg) therapy in infected newborn babies*

	Antibiotics ($n=15$)		Antibiotics plus IVIg ($n=20$)	
	Total no.	No. died	Total no.	No. died
Gestation				
<38 weeks	9	4	13	1 (*P* 0.04)
>38 weeks	6	0	7	1
Birthweight				
<2500 g	9	4	11	1
>2500 g	6	0	9	1
Total	15	4	20	2 (*P* 0.16)

From Sidiropoulous et al. (34).

Table 10.2. *Results of prophylactic intravenous immunoglobulin therapy in preterm and low-birthweight infants*

	Total no.	No. (and %) infected	No. (and %) infected
Group A	50	2 (4)	0
Group B	50	2 (4)	0
Control	50	8 (16)	2 (4)†

*$P<0.005$; †$P<0.001$.

Reproduced from KN Haque et al. (41), Intravenous immunoglobulin for prevention of sepsis in preterm and low birth weight infants, Pediatr Infect Dis, 5, 622–5, ©by Williams & Wilkins, 1986.

increased susceptibility to infection, suppression of cellular response (bacille Calmette-Guérin (BCG) vaccination), depression of endogenous immunoglobulin production or response to routine immunization.

Several commercial IVIg preparations have been tested for their protective efficacy. Fischer et al. (39) have shown that gammaglobulin modified by reduction and alkylation decreased mortality in suckling rats from sepsis due to type Ia, II and III strains of GBS. Christensen et al. (40) have reported that gammaglobulin preparations, prepared by mild acid treatment (pH 4.0), gave adult mice protection from lethal GBS infection with type Ia, II and III strains.

Encouraged by the results of the studies referred to above, we wondered whether passive IVIg therapy would prevent sepsis and reduce mortality in a high-risk population of low-birthweight (LBW) and preterm infants. In a randomized prospective trial of prophylactic IVIg administration in preterm and LBW infants we found (41) a highly significant reduction in the rate of infections and a significant decrease in the mortality rate from neonatal sepsis (Table 10.2). In this study the effect of a polyvalent IVIg preparation given prophylactically to prevent neonatal sepsis was tested in preterm and LBW infants. Infants matched for gestational age, sex, and birthweight within 250-g groups were randomly allocated into three groups of 50 each, one group (group C) being used as control.

Group A received Intraglobin® (Biotest Pharma, Frankfurt, West Germany), 120 mg/kg intravenously within 2–4 h of birth; group B received the same on days 1 and 8. The control group received no immunoglobulin. The frequency of infection, outcome and serum immunoglobulin concentrations were determined in each group. Infection rate in the control group was 16% (8/50), while in each of the treated groups it was 4% (2/50, $P<0.05$). There were no deaths in the two treated groups, while in the control group, two (4%) infants died ($P<0.001$). The serum immunoglobulin concentrations achieved in the treated groups were significantly higher than in the control group (Figs 10.1–10.3). Interestingly, after IVIg infusion not only did serum IgG rise ninefold in the treated groups but IgM also rose sixfold in these two groups. A similar increase in serum IgG levels was reported by Sidiropolous et al. (54), but the rise in serum IgM remains unexplained. It may be due to increased antigenic recognition stimulated by IVIg or to the impurities in the preparation acting as antigens. However, it is possible that, by overcoming the transitory lack of IgM

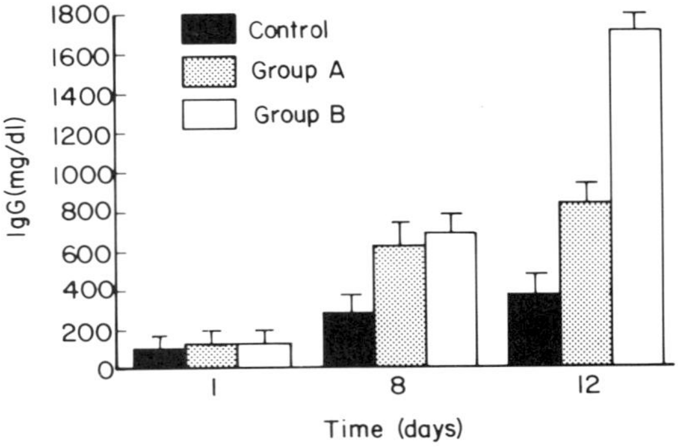

Fig. 10.1. Serum IgG concentrations. Difference in the mean values between days 1, 8 and 12: Group A, $P<0.001$; Group B, $P<0.001$; control, P non-significant. Student's *t*-test. Bars indicate SD. Reproduced from KN Haque et al. (41), Intravenous immunoglobulin for prevention of sepsis in preterm and low birth weight infants, Pediatr Infect Dis, 5, 662–5, ©by Williams & Wilkins, 1986.

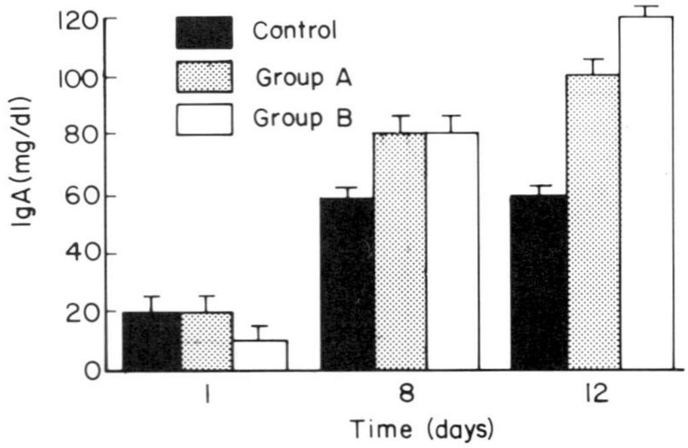

Fig. 10.2. Serum IgA concentrations. Difference in the mean values between days 1, 8 and 12: Group A, $P<0.005$; Group B, $P<0.001$. Control group difference between days 1 and 8, $P<0.005$; days 8 and 12, P non-significant. Student's *t*-test. Bars indicate SD. Reproduced from KN Haque et al. (41), Intravenous immunoglobulin for prevention of sepsis in preterm and low birth weight infants, Pediatr Infect Dis, 5, 662–5, ©by Williams & Wilkins, 1986.

in these infants (42), the rise in IgM was responsible for the favourable outcome of our study.

There are many theoretical reasons why boosting serum IgM in the newborn would help the infant to combat sepsis:

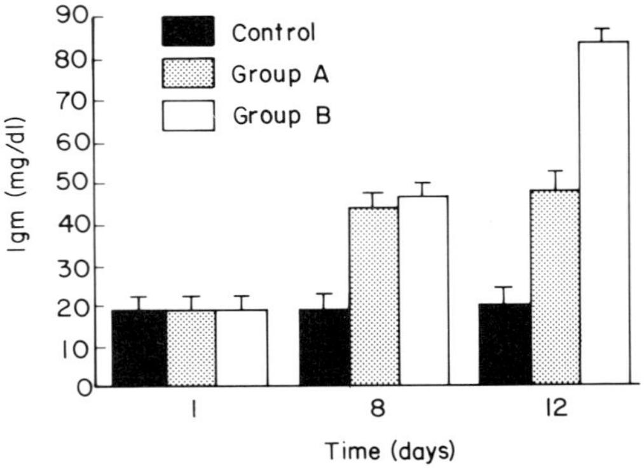

Fig. 10.3. Serum IgM concentrations. Difference in the mean values between days 1, 8 and 12: Group A, $P<0.001$; Group B, $P<0.001$; control, P non-significant. Student's *t*-test. Bars indicate SD. Reproduced from KN Haque et al. (41), Intravenous immunoglobulin for prevention of sepsis in preterm and low birth weight infants, Pediatr Infect Dis, 5, 662–5, ©by Williams & Wilkins, 1986.

(1) IgM is the first specific antibody response (13);
(2) IgM requires a less extensive cascade of cooperating cells and factors than does IgG;
(3) IgM has the ability to fix complement and thus enhance opsonization;
(4) IgM can alter cell-wall characteristics of antigen (43), initiating its lysis or intracellular lysis after phagocytosis.

We thus decided to study the effect of IgM-enriched IVIg in the treatment of neonatal sepsis.

Two groups of 30 preterm infants with sepsis were studied. They were matched for gestational age, sex, birthweight and Apgar score (Table 10.3). Only infants with their first episode of sepsis were enrolled in the study. The criteria used in this study for diagnosis of sepsis are shown in Table 10.4. Whenever sepsis was suspected, an infant was randomly allocated either to a control group who received supportive therapy (correction of fluid, acid–base balance, nutrition, good

Table 10.3. *IgM-enriched immunoglobulin study: basic data for the two groups*

	No.	Gestational age (weeks)	Birthweight (kg)	Male/female ratio	Mean Apgar score at 5 min	SGA	PROM
Controls	30	28–37 (35)*	0.9–1.7 (1.48)	20/10	7	2	4
Immunotherapy group	30	28–37 (33.4)	0.85–1.6 (1.32)	24/6	7	1	5

*Means are given in parentheses.

SGA, small for gestational age; PROM, prolonged rupture of membranes (>24 h).

Table 10.4. *Criteria for diagnosis of neonatal sepsis IgM-enriched immunoglobulin study:*

Clinical signs	Laboratory tests
Lethargy	WBC <5000/μl
Instability of temperature	WBC >30 000/μl
	I/T >0.2
Glucose intolerance	Platelet count <50 000/μl
Increasing gastric residue	Positive blood culture
Hepatosplenomegaly	Positive CSF culture

WBC, white blood cell count; I/T immature/total neutrophils; CSF, cerebrospinal fluid.

Whenever either the blood or the CSF culture was positive, the case was considered as *proven sepsis*. When clinical features were present but cultures were negative, the case was considered as *suspected sepsis*.

thermal environment) plus ampicillin 100 mg/kg/24 h and gentamicin 3 mg/kg/24 h, or to an immunotherapy group who received the same as above plus 5 ml/kg/24 h intravenous IgM-enriched immunoglobulin (Pentaglobin®, Biotest Pharma, Frankfurt, West German), given over 2 h on days 1–4 inclusive. Before instituting any therapy in either group, full investigations for infection were carried out. Blood was also taken for serum immunoglobulin assay on days 1, 7 and 10. For the purposes of analysis the two groups were further divided into cases of *proven sepsis*, when cultures were positive, and cases of *suspected sepsis*, when cultures were negative and the diagnosis was based on clinical criteria alone.

There were 21 cases of *proven sepsis* and nine of *suspected sepsis* in the immunotherapy group, while in the control group there were 23 cases of *proven sepsis* and seven of *suspected sepsis*. The number of infections, causative organisms and the outcome in each group are shown in Table 10.5. Applying Student's *t*-test, there was a significant difference in the outcome of the two groups: six (20%) infants died in the control group, while in the immunotherapy group only one (3%) infant died ($P<0.001$). *Escherichia coli* was the most frequent organism to be isolated, being responsible for 43% of infections in the control group and 38% in the immunotherapy group (44).

Serum immunoglobulin levels are shown in Figs 10.4–10.6. There was a significant rise in serum IgM and IgA in the immunotherapy group; IgG also rose in both groups, but the difference did not achieve statistical significance. The total white blood cell count and the immature to total neutrophil ratio returned to normal earlier in the immunotherapy group than in the control group, but again the difference was not statistically significant. However, fewer infants in the immunotherapy group developed neutropenia – a feature frequently associated with poorer outcome (45).

Although no major complications have been reported to date when IVIg preparations are infused slowly, the results and complications have significant lot-to-lot variability, particularly in the concentration of functional type-specific antibody. For this reason it should be noted that the clinical results

Table 10.5. *IgM-enriched immunoglobulin study: number of infections, causative organisms and outcome*

	No. of infections	Organisms (and no. of cases)	Mortality	%
Control group				
Proven sepsis	23	*Escherichia coli* (10)		
		Klebsiella pneumoniae (5)	4	
		Salmonella spp. (4)		20
		Staphylococcus epidermidis (3)		
		Serratia spp. (1)		
Suspected sepsis	7		2	
Immunotherapy group				
Proven sepsis	21	*Escherichia coli* (8)		
		Klebsiella pneumoniae (6)	1	
		Staphylococcus epidermidis (2)		3.3
		Salmonella spp. (3)		
		Serratia spp. (1)		
		Pseudomonas aeruginosa (1)		
Suspected sepsis	9		0	

$^{*}P<0.001$.

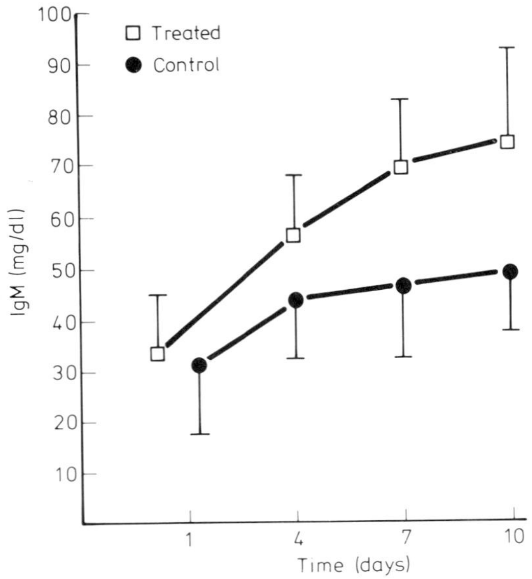

Fig. 10.4. Serum IgM concentrations. Difference in the mean values between the two groups on days 7 and 10: $P<0.001$. Student's *t*-test. Bars indicate SD.

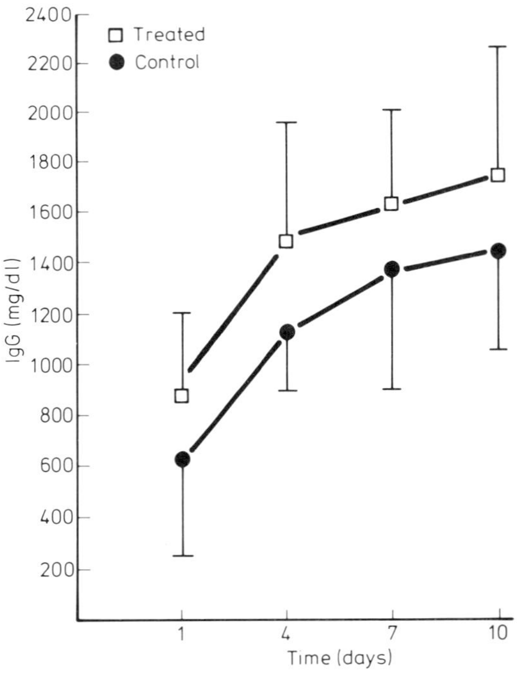

Fig. 10.5. Serum IgG concentrations. Difference in the mean values between the two groups was not significant. Student's *t*-test. Bars indicate SD.

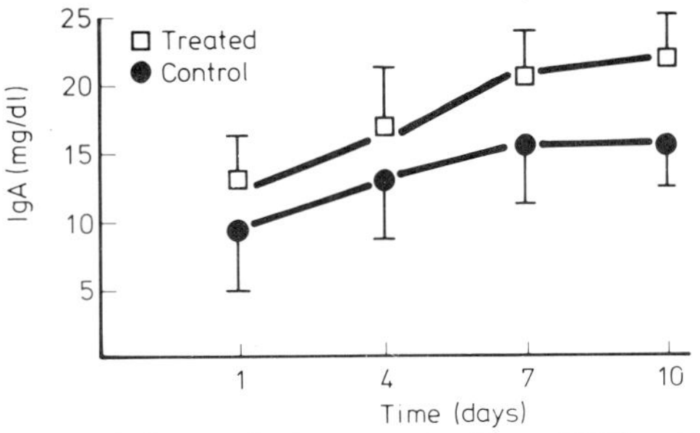

Fig. 10.6. Serum IgA concentrations. Difference in the mean values on day 10: $P<0.01$. Student's *t*-test. Bars indicate SD.

obtained with one IVIg preparation cannot be used to estimate the efficacy of another preparation. The biological properties depend on the manufacturing processes (45). These, while trying to avoid anticomplement and prekallikrein activity, may alter the structure of the gammaglobulin molecule, thus changing its biological activity, for example the opsonic effect. This difference in the gammaglobulin may be responsible for the lack of effect of IVIg in neonatal sepsis reported by Stabile et al. (46). The largest study to date has been conducted by Chirico et al. (47), who selected alternate infants weighing 1500 g or less for treatment with 0.5 g/kg/week IVIg for 4 weeks. Thirty-one of 40 (77%) infants in the group who did not receive IVIg developed infection and 13 (32%) died, while of the 43 receiving IVIg, only 22 (51%) developed infection and seven (16%) died.

Table 10.6. *Gammaglobulin preparations*

Product name	Manufacturer	Treatment of preparation during manufacturing process
1. Endobulin	Immuno AG, Vienna, Austria	Polyethylene glycol treatment and isoelectric precipitation
2. Immunoglobulin Human 7 S	Armour Pharma, West Germany	Polyethylene glycol and hydroxyethyl starch treatment
3. Sandoglobulin	Sandoz AG, West Germany	pH-4 treatment with traces of pepsin
4. Intraglobin	Biotest GmbH, West Germany	Beta-propiolactone treatment
5. Human Gammaglobulin	Merieux SA, Lyon, France	Plasmin degradation
6. Intact Intravenous Immunoglobulin	Merieux SA, Lyon, France	Polyethylene glycol treatment
7. Gamma-Venin	Behring Werke, West Germany	Pepsin degradation
8. Venimmun	Behring Werke, West Germany	Limited sulphitolysis
9. Polyglobulin Cutter	Troponwerke, West Germany	Reduction and alkylation
10. IVIG Cutter	Cutter Laboratories, California, USA	Reduction and alkylation
11. Gammantiv	Kabi Vitrum AB, Stockholm, Sweden	DEAE sephadex A50 chrom-stabilized with human albumin
12. Menselijk Normaal Immunoglobuline	Netherland Red Cross, Amsterdam, The Netherlands	pH-4 treatment with traces of pepsin

DEAE, diethylaminoethyl.
All preparations made by cold-ethanol fractionation of blood plasma, except Human Gammaglobulin and Intact Intravenous Immunoglobulin, which are both isolated from human placenta.

From van Furth et al. (48), with permission.

van Furth et al. (48) have studied 12 different commercial IVIg preparations (Table 10.6). A significant correlation was found between the concentration of intact IgG molecules in each batch and the opsonic activity; the preparations which showed little opsonic activity were the ones which had decreased quantities of intact IgG molecules. They also found after ultracentrifugation that almost all preparations contained aggregates, but the highest proportion of IgG fragmentation was seen in preparations from Human Gammaglobulin® and Gamma-Venin®, both of which are enzyme-treated preparations. On the basis of their study the authors concluded that IVIg preparations produced by Immuno AG, Armour Pharma, Sandoz AG, Biotest GmbH, Merieux SA (Intact Intravenous Immunoglobulin), Behring Werke (Venimmun), Kabi Vitrum AB and Netherlands Red Cross showed good opsonic activity.

For years immunoglobulins manufactured by Cohn fractionation were considered to be safe from transmission of viruses. However, some recent publications (49–53) show that non-A, non-B hepatitis may be transmitted by use of IVIg. Preparations treated by beta-propiolactone, such as Intraglobin®, eliminate this risk.

Conclusion

Our work and other reports indicate that we have just begun to tap the potential uses of IVIg. Although questions remain about the dosage, frequency and duration of IVIg therapy, there is very little doubt that IVIg is a major advance in the treatment of neonatal sepsis. We (41, 44) have shown that IgG preparations are best suited for prevention, whereas IgM-enriched preparations should be used in the treatment of neonatal sepsis. We hope that further studies will be conducted to confirm our work and the work of Eible et al. (54), who have shown the preventive effect of oral IgA-enriched immunoglobulin in the prevention of necrotizing enterocolitis.

References

1. Hill HR. Diagnosis and treatment of sepsis in the neonate: septic shock. In: Root Contemporary issues in infectious diseases, vol. 4.
2. Santos JI, Hill HR. Bacterial infection of the neonate. In: Wedgwood RJ, Davis SD, Ray CG et al. (eds), Infections in children. Philadelphia: Harper and Row, 1982: 179–202.
3. Hill HR. Group B streptococcal infections. In: Holmes KK, Mardh PA, Sparling PF, et al. (eds), Sexually transmitted disease. New York: McGraw-Hill, 1984: 397–407.
4. Klein JO, Marcy SM. Bacterial sepsis and meningitis. In: Remington JS, Klein JO (eds), Infectious diseases of the fetus and the newborn infant. Philadelphia: WB Saunders, 1983: 679–735.
5. Hemming VG, Hall RT, Rhodes PG et al. Assessment of group B streptococcal opsonins in human and rabbit serum by neutrophil chemiluminescence. J Clin Invest 1976; 58: 1379–87.
6. Baker CJ, Kasper DL. Correlation of maternal antibody deficiency with susceptibility to neonatal group B streptococcal infection. N Engl J Med 1976; 294: 752–6.
7. Dossett JH, Williams RC Jr, Quie PG. Studies on interaction of bacteria serum factors and polymorphonuclear leukocytes in mothers and newborns. Pediatrics 1969; 44: 49–57.
8. Ballow M, Fang F, Good RA et al. Developmental aspects of complement components in the newborn. Clin Exp Immunol 1974; 18: 257–66.
9. Hill HR, Hogan NA, Bale JF et al. Evaluation of non specific (alternate pathway) opsonic activity by neutrophil chemiluminescence. Int Arch Allergy Appl Immunol 1977; 53: 490–7.
10. Shigeoka AO, Jensen C, Pincus SH et al. Absolute requirement for complement in IgM mediated protection against experimental type III group B streptococcal infection. J Infect Dis 1984; 150: 63–70.
11. Hill HR. Host defences in the neonate: prospects for enhancement. Semin Perinatol 1985; 9: 2–11.
12. Barnard DR, Arthur MM. Fibronectin (cold insoluble globulin) in the neonate. J Pediatr 1983; 102: 453–5.

13. Harper TE, Christensen RD, Rothstein G et al. Effect of intravenous immunoglobulin G on neutrophil kinetics during experimental group B streptococcal infection in neonatal rats. Rev Infect Dis 1986; 8(suppl): S401–8.
14. Sacchi F, Hill HR. Defective membrane potential changes in neutrophils from human neonates. J Exp Med 1984; 160: 1247–52.
15. Christensen RD, Macfarlane JL, Taylor NL et al. Blood and marrow neutrophils during experimental group B streptococcal infection: quantification of stem cell, proliferative, storage and circulating pools. Pediatr Res 1982; 16: 549–53.
16. Christensen RD, Hill HR, Rothstein G. Granulocyte stem cell (CFUc) proliferation in experimental group B streptococcal sepsis. Pediatr Res 1983; 17: 278–80.
17. Ohlsson A, Serenius F. Neonatal septicemia in Riyadh, Saudi Arabia. Acta Paediatr Scand 1981; 70: 825–9.
18. el Rifai MR. A study of 214 neonates with infection in Maternity and Childrens Hospital, Riyadh, Saudi Arabia. Ann Trop Paediatr 1982; 3: 19–22.
19. Oto A. Major bacterial infections in a referral neonatal intensive care unit. J Infect 1982; 5: 117–26.
20. Freedman RM, Ingram DL, Gross I et al. A half century of neonatal sepsis at Yale. Am J Dis Child 1981; 135: 140–5.
21. Steen JA, Gammaglobulin in preventing infections in premature infants. Arch Paediatr 1960; 77: 291–4.
22. Amer J, Olt E, Ibbolt FA et al. The effect of monthly gammaglobulin administration on morbidity and mortality from infection in premature infants during first year of life. Pediatrics 1963; 32: 4–9.
23. Morell A, Skvaril F, van Loghem E et al. Human IgG subclass in maternal and fetal serum. Vox Sang 1971; 21: 481–92.
24. Evans HE, Akpata SO, Glass L. Serum immunoglobulin levels in premature and full term infants. Pediatr Infect Dis 1986; 5: 620–1.
25. Wasserman RL. Intravenous gammaglobulin prophylaxis for newborn infants. Pediatr Infect Dis 1986; 5: 620–1.
26. Christensen RD. Morphology and concentration of circulating neutrophils in neonates with bacterial sepsis. Pediatr Infect Dis 1987; 6: 429–30.
27. Akenzua GI, Hui YT, Milner R et al. Neutrophil and band counts in the diagnosis of neonatal infection. Pediatrics 1974; 54: 38–42.
28. Philips AGS, Hewitt JR. Early diagnosis of neonatal sepsis. Pediatrics 1980; 65: 1036–41.
29. Manroe BL, Rosenfield CR, Weinberg AG et al. Differential leukocyte count in assessment of outcome of early-onset neonatal group B streptococcal disease. J Pediatr 1977; 91: 632–7.
30. Liu CH, Lethan C, Speer ME et al. Degenerative changes in neutrophils: an indicator of bacterial infection. Pediatrics 1984; 74: 823–7.
31. Fischer GW, Weismann LB, Hemming VG et al. Intravenous immunoglobulin in neonatal group B streptococcal disease. Am J Med 1984; 76: 117–23.
32. Yoder MC, Polin RA. Immunotherapy of neonatal septicemia. Ped Clin North Am 1986; 33: 481–501.
33. Harper TE, Christensen RD, Rothstein G et al. The effect of administration of IgG to newborn rats with *E. coli* sepsis and meningitis. Ped Res 1987; 22: 455–60.
34. Sidiropolous D, Bhome U, von Murait G et al. Immunoglobulin substitution in the treatment of neonatal sepsis. Schweiz Med Wochensch 1981; 111: 1649–55.
35. Fischer GW, Hemming VG, Hunter KW et al. Intravenous immunoglobulin in the treatment of neonatal sepsis: therapeutic strategies and laboratory studies. Pediatr Infect Dis (suppl) 1986; 5(3): S171–5.
36. Weismann LE, Fischer GW, Hemming VG, Peck CC. Pharmacokinetics of intravenous immunoglobulin (Sandoglobulin) in neonates. Pediatr Infect Dis (suppl) 1986; 5(3): S185–8.
37. Christensen KK, Christensen P. Intravenous gammaglobulin in the treatment of neonatal sepsis with special reference to group B streptococci and pharmacokinetics. Pediatr Infect Dis (suppl) 1986; 5(3) S189–92.
38. Morell A, Sidiropolous D, Herrmann U et al. IgG subclasses and antibodies to group B streptococci in preterm neonates after intravenous infusion of immunoglobulin to the mothers. Pediatr Infect Dis (suppl) 1986; 5(3): S195–7.
39. Fischer GW, Hunter KW, Wilson SR. Modified human serum globulin for intravenous administration: *in vitro* opsonic activity and *in vivo* protection against group B streptococcal disease in suckling rats. Acta Paediatr Scand 1982; 71: 639–44.
40. Christensen KK, Christensen P, Duc G et al. Human IgG antibodies to carbohydrate and protein antigens in mouse protection tests with group B streptococci. Pediatr Res 1984; 18: 478–82.

41. Haque KN, Zaidi MH, Haque SK et al. Intravenous immunoglobulin for prevention of sepsis in preterm and low birth weight infants. Pediatr Infect Dis 1986; 5: 622–5.
42. van Furth R, Schutt HRE, Hijmans W. The immunological development of human fetus. J Exp Med 1965; 122: 1173–88.
43. Stubner G. Indirect evidence of cell wall alterations in *Pseudomonas aeruginosa* by immunoglobulin preparations. Infection 1984; 12: 223–4.
44. Haque KN, Zaidi MH, Bahakim H. IgM-enriched intravenous immunoglobulin therapy in neonatal sepsis. Am J Dis Child 1988; 142: 1293–6.
45. Squire E, Favara B, Todd J. Diagnosis of neonatal bacterial infection: hematologic and pathologic findings in fatal and non fatal cases. Pediatrics 1979; 64: 60–4.
46. Stabile A, Sopos SM, Romanelli V et al. Intravenous immunoglobulin for prophylaxis of neonatal sepsis in preterm infants. Am J Dis Child 1988; 63: 441–3.
47. Chirico G, Rondini G, Pelbani A et al. Intravenous gammaglobulin therapy for prophylaxis of infection in high risk neonates. J Pediatr 1987; 110: 437–42.
48. van Furth R, Leijh PCJ, Klein F. Correlation between opsonic activities for various microorganisms and composition of gammaglobulin preparations for intravenous use. J Infect Dis 1984; 149: 511–17.
49. Ochs HD, Fisher S, Virant FS et al. Non A non B hepatitis and intravenous immunoglobulins. Lancet 1985; 1: 404–5.
50. Lane RS. Non A non B hepatitis from intravenous immunoglobulins. Lancet 1983; 2: 974–5.
51. Lever AML, Webster ADB, Brown D et al. Non A non B hepatitis occurring in agammaglobunemic patients after intravenous immunoglobulin. Lancet 1984; 2: 1062–4.
52. Welch AG, Cuthbertson B, McIntosh RV et al. Non A non B hepatitis from intravenous immunoglobulin. Lancet 1983; 2: 1198–9.
53. Stephan W, Dichtelmuller H. Non A non B hepatitis from intravenous immunoglobulins. Lancet 1983; 2: 1488.
54. Eible MM, Herman M, Wolf MD et al. Prevention of necrotizing enterocolitis in low-birth-weight infants by IgA-IgG feeding. N Engl J Med 1988; 319: 1–7.

11 Antibiotic Policies

M. A. Hall
Princess Anne Hospital and
Southampton General Hospital,
Southampton, UK

Introduction

Almost from the moment of their introduction as therapeutic agents antibiotics have assumed a major role in the first-line management of sick newborn infants. Despite many early misadventures, which have been well described elsewhere (1), most neonatologists would agree that the potential benefits of early, and possibly unnecessary, antibiotic treatment outweigh the risks inherent in such a policy. Over the past few years many units have witnessed an increase in the proportion of bacterial isolates which have become resistant to the commonly used antibiotics, while doubts have been expressed about the safety of both established and new chemotherapeutic agents. The purpose of this chapter is to review the way in which antibiotics are used in neonatology and to discuss the advantages and disadvantages of some of the various regimens currently available.

Antibiotics and sepsis in current neonatal practice

The extent of antibiotic prescribing in neonatal units

Antibiotics are administered to newborn infants for a variety of reasons, parenterally to treat suspected septicaemia, pneumonia or meningitis and topically to treat conditions such as conjunctivitis, thrush and omphalitis. In addition, many units apply a topical antiseptic to the normal umbilical cord stump until separation has occurred. There have been few published reports concerning the extent of antibiotic usage, but it is probable that the majority of babies who receive intensive care during the newborn period are prescribed parenteral broad-spectrum antibiotics at some time during their admission (2). In the mid-1970s a study from Boston in the USA reported that 4.4% of all babies born in a hospital serving a middle-class population

Table 11.1. *Frequency of parenteral antibiotic treatment in neonates*

Hospital (Ref. no.)	Year	No. of live births	No. treated with antibiotics	% treated
Hospital A Boston (3)	1977	1011	44	4.4
Hospital B Boston (3)	1977	540	57	10.6
Princess Anne Southampton (4)	1986	5273	160	3.0

Infection in the Newborn. Edited by J. de Louvois and D. Harvey
©1990 John Wiley & Sons Ltd

(Hospital A) received parenteral antibiotics – in most cases an aminoglycoside and penicillin – compared to 10.6% of babies born in a hospital serving a poorer inner-city population (Hospital B) (3). Only 6.8% and 3.5% respectively of those treated were found to have positive blood cultures. In 1986 in Southampton, England, 3.0% of all babies born during the year received parenteral broad-spectrum antibiotics (Table 11.1) and 0.5 received more than one such course (4).

Bacterial causes of neonatal sepsis

The bacteria which cause early sepsis – sepsis occurring within the first 2 or 3 days of life – are usually quite different from those giving rise to sepsis later in the neonatal period (5, 6). Early bacterial sepsis is usually caused by organisms which are acquired from the maternal genital tract and which have not developed the patterns of antibiotic resistance often seen in those isolated from older neonates (7). In some areas *Staphylococcus aureus* and *Listeria monocytogenes* are also important causes of early neonatal sepsis (8). Organisms which cause late sepsis – after the first few days of life – include *Staphylococcus epidermidis*, *Staph. aureus*, *Klebsiella* sp., *Enterbacter* sp., *Pseudomonas* sp., and other coliforms which are acquired from the nursery environment and whose antibiotic sensitivities have been influenced by prevailing practices. Thus there are good reasons for having separate antibiotic policies for early and late suspected sepsis.

While the fulminating nature and high mortality rate associated with early group B streptococcal infection are often stressed, the outcome from early gram-negative sepsis, particularly from that caused by *Escherichia coli*, can be equally poor. The clinical signs of neonatal sepsis are notoriously non-specific (5, 9) and septic infants can become moribund within an hour or two of appearing to be only mildly unwell.

Postnatal age and antibiotic prescribing

The majority of neonates who receive parenteral antibiotics do so within the first 2 or 3 days of life. In the Boston study 95% of infants in Hospital A and 91% in Hospital B started their treatment during the first 3 days of life. Similarly, in a combined randomized study of antibiotic treatment of suspected neonatal sepsis involving the Special Care Baby Units in Chatham, England, and Southampton (4) it was found that 89% of the Chatham babies who received parenteral antibiotics and 94% of those in Southampton started their treatment within 3 days of birth. Thus, in current clinical practice, blind antibiotic treatment is most commonly used soon after birth. Although antibiotics are frequently used in older babies, they may be more specifically selected to cover conditions such as necrotizing enterocolitis or organisms of known antibiotic sensitivity such as *Staph. epidermidis* or *Pseudomonas* sp.

In particular, it is well known that early-onset group B streptococcal sepsis usually presents with signs of respiratory difficulties, often indistinguishable from those seen in the idiopathic respiratory-distress syndrome (7, 10). It is inevitable, therefore, that many babies who are not infected will receive antibiotic treatment.

The diagnosis of bacterial sepsis in the newborn

The proportion of treated babies whose clinical signs prove to be attributable to infection is, in fact, extremely small. In Table 11.2 it can be seen that the yield of positive blood or cerebrospinal fluid (CSF) cultures was extremely low in a selection of studies reported over the past 10 years. However, some infants with negative blood and CSF cultures in these studies were reported to be suffering from bacterial sepsis on the basis of their clinical signs and

Table 11.2. *Positive deep cultures in suspected neonatal sepsis*

Hospital (Ref. no)	Year	No. of episodes of suspected sepsis*	% of episodes in which blood/CSF culture +ve
Hospital A Boston (3)	1977	44	7
Hospital B Boston (3)	1977	57	3.5
Hammersmith London (11)	1983	70	4.3
Dudley Road Birmingham (12)	1985	108	11
Queen Charlotte's London (13)	1985	446	4.5

*Only babies treated with antibiotics included.

CSF, cerebrospinal fluid.

Table 11.3. *Classification of infection in neonates treated for suspected sepsis*

Hospital (Ref. no)	Year	No. treated	Proven or definite sepsis	Very probable or probable sepsis
Medical Center Vermont (14)	1980	328	30 (9%)	20 (6%)
All Saints Chatham (4)	1986	123	5 (4%)	19 (15%)
Princess Anne Southampton (4)	1986	99	3 (3%)	15 (15%)

peripheral swab cultures, and such infants must be taken into account when assessing the use of antibiotics in neonates. In an attempt to identify neonates who are infected but who have negative blood and CSF cultures, Philip and Hewitt (14) showed that the use of certain simple laboratory tests could help in determining whether infants were likely to be infected. Our own combined study in Chatham and Southampton used a modification of their protocol and the results of all three studies are shown in Table 11.3.

From these, and other, observations it would seem reasonable to conclude that, in the treatment of *suspected* neonatal sepsis:

(1) most antibiotic courses are started within 3 days of birth;
(2) the commonly identified infecting organisms isolated within the first 3 days are not hospital-acquired;
(3) a large majority of those infants who are treated are not actually infected.

In the Chatham/Southampton study, despite the fact that more than 80% of treated babies were not infected, 57% received antibiotic treatment for 4 or more days. In view of the large numbers of newborn infants who receive blind antibiotic treatment for suspected neonatal sepsis and of the relatively low rate of infection, it is of paramount importance that the chemotherapeutic agents which are selected not only should be highly effective for the few babies who turn out to be suffering from systemic bacterial infection, but also should be shown to have no, or minimal, adverse effects.

Antibiotic options for the treatment of early sepsis

The aminoglycosides

The subject of antibiotic treatment in the newborn has been reviewed in at least three recent publications (5, 15, 16). The proven track record of the combination of an aminoglycoside with penicillin or ampicillin is indisputable; at present this must be regarded as the gold standard of chemotherapeutic choice, at least for the management of suspected early sepsis. Nevertheless, the implications of such a policy do warrant further consideration.

Clinical problems associated with aminoglycosides

There can be little doubt that a penicillin plus aminoglycoside combination provides good cover against the organisms which are likely to cause early sepsis. There are, however, well recognized problems associated with the use of these compounds in older patients and some of these are listed in Table 11.4. The main uncertainties concern the potential toxicity of the aminoglycosides. Of the adverse effects, ototoxicity is probably the most important since, at least in animal and adult studies, the ensuing cochlear or vestibular damage is usually irreversible. Several authors have referred to the lack of evidence to implicate aminoglycoside treatment as a numerically important cause of hearing impairment resulting from the neonatal period (15, 17, 18) and, in a recent authoritative review of aminoglycoside toxicity in the newborn, McCracken has summarized the evidence currently available (19). It is clear that deafness attributable to aminoglycosides is, indeed, uncommon but few would claim that it *never* occurs and several of the quoted studies have cited individual cases in which deafness has been thought to be due to aminoglycoside toxicity (19, 20). The difficulties and methodological problems inherent in most of the studies are well known and it is likely that, in view of the large numbers which would be required for a definitive study, the true risk of deafness resulting from treatment of the newborn with aminoglycosides will never be known (21).

Table 11.4. *Disadvantages of the aminoglycosides*

Ototoxicity
Nephrotoxicity
Neuromuscular blockade
Poor CSF penetration
Variable pulmonary penetration
Need to monitor blood levels

CSF, cerebrospinal fluid.

The second major unwanted effect is nephrotoxicity. Aminoglycoside-induced abnormalities of tubular function have been shown in several studies of mainly low-birthweight infants (22–24), but no long-term adverse effects have been documented. Glomerular dysfunction associated with gentamicin treatment was also reported recently (25). Both animal and human studies have indicated that, unlike the ototoxicity, aminoglycoside nephrotoxicity is usually fully reversible, but the extent to which such transient changes in tubular or glomerular function affect the clinical course of sick neonates is not known. Interactions between the aminoglycosides and commonly used drugs such as frusemide (26) and indomethacin (27) may also be important in the newborn.

The aminoglycoside antibiotics are known to have a potential neuromuscular blocking action (28), which may, rarely, be associated with postanaesthetic respiratory paralysis. In the newborn there have been isolated reports of neuromuscular blockade associated with aminoglycoside administration to infants with botulism (29) and hypermagnesaemia (30), but this effect has not been the subject of extensive detailed studies in low-birthweight babies.

A further potential limitation of aminoglycoside antibiotics is their relatively poor ability to cross biological membranes (31), giving rise to some doubts about their efficacy in the treatment of bacterial meningitis and infections of the lung. In neonates, however, any such concerns have been regarded by most authorities as theoretical, and an aminoglycoside plus ampicillin is the treatment of choice, on empirical grounds, for neonatal meningitis in many hospitals (32). In addition, there have been reports of relatively high levels of both gentamicin and netilmicin in the lungs of treated newborn infants at autopsy (33, 34), indicating that concerns about poor lung penetration of these antibiotics in adults may not be relevant to the newborn.

More compelling, perhaps, is the evidence from studies of older patients treated with aminoglycosides. In a survey of 144 clinical trials published between 1975 and 1982 and covering almost 10 000 patients – mainly adults or older children – Kahlmeter and Dahlager calculated the average frequencies of toxic effects attributed to four of the commonly used aminoglycosides (35). Their findings are shown in Table 11.5.

While many of the studies included in this survey are likely to have overestimated the frequency of adverse effects, it must be concluded that such sequelae are relatively common, if only transiently. It is unlikely, therefore, that the concerns of many neonatologists about aminoglycoside toxicity will be completely dispelled by the results of clinical trials, despite the fact that serious adverse effects must be uncommon. Certainly, blood-level monitoring is regarded as mandatory and dosage adjustments are frequently made as a result, leading to further blood-level measurements. In our own study, dosage was changed in 31% of patients receiving netilmicin compared to only 3% of those receiving a third-generation cephalosporin (4).

Table 11.5. *Nephrotoxicity and ototoxicity resulting from aminoglycoside treatment in older patients*

	Renal toxicity (%)*	Cochlear toxicity (%)	Vestibular toxicity (%)
Gentamicin	14.0	8.3	3.2
Tobramycin	12.9	6.1	3.5
Netilmicin	8.7	2.4	1.4
Amikacin	9.4	13.9	2.8

*Percentage of treated patients.

Data from Kahlmeter and Dahlager (35).

In order to minimize the risk imposed by antibiotic treatment of the newborn, it would seem reasonable to consider the following questions:

(1) If a combination of aminoglycoside plus penicillin/ampicillin is to be used as first-line treatment of suspected neonatal sepsis, which of the aminoglycosides is the safest and most effective?
(2) Are there safe and effective alternatives to the aminoglycoside plus penicillin/ampicillin combination?

Which aminoglycoside?

The main considerations in selecting any medication for use in newborn infants are those of safety and efficacy. In view of the lack of documented long-term toxicity, it could be argued that the theoretical side-effects need not be a major factor in deciding which one to use. For those concerned about the possible harmful effects, however, there is evidence from animal and human studies that netilmicin is associated with the lowest rates of both nephro- and ototoxicity (18, 35–37) (Table 11.5). There have been few comparative toxicity studies in human neonates (20, 22).

Although all of the aminoglycosides have a wide range of activity against aerobic bacteria, particularly against gram-negative organisms, there are some intrinsic differences between them. Gentamicin and tobramycin

Table 11.6. *Antibacterial spectra of cephalosporins*

	Cephalo-ridine	Cephalo-thin	Cefacetrile	Cefazolin	Cephoglycin	Cephalexin	Cephradine	Cefatrizine	Cefadroxil	Cefachlor	Cefamandole	Cefoxitin	Cefuroxime	Cefotaxime
Staphylococcus aureus	0.25	0.5	1	0.25	2	2	2	0.5	2	4	0.5	4	1	2
Staphylococcus aureus penicillinase positive	4	0.5	2	2	4	2	2	2	4	8	2	4	1	2
Streptococcus pyogenes	0.01	0.12	0.5	0.25	0.12	0.5	0.5	0.12	0.5	0.25	0.12	0.5	0.03	0.06
Streptococcus faecalis	16	32	16	R	R	R	R	R	R	R	32	R	R	2
Streptococcus pneumoniae	0.03	0.06	0.25	0.12	0.25	2	2	0.5	1.0	1.0	0.25	1.0	0.03	
Neisseria gonorrhoeae	0.25	0.25		0.12		0.5	0.5	0.25		0.12		0.25	0.06	0.001
Haemophilus influenzae	8	8		8	16	32	32	8	32	2	2	4	0.5	0.03
Escherichia coli	4	8	8	4	2	8	16	8	16	8	4	4	4	0.1
Klebsiella sp.	4	4	8	4	2	8	16	8	16	8	2	4	4	0.1
Enterobacter sp.	R	R	R	R	R	R	R	R	R	R	R	R	8	0.1–R
Proteus mirabilis	4	4	8	4	2	16	16	8	16	16	2	4	4	0.06
Proteus sp., indole positive	R	R	R	R	R	R	R	R	R	R	R	8	8	0.2–2
Serratia sp.	R	R	R	R	R	R	R	R	R	R	R	16	8	0.5
Salmonella sp.	2	2	8	2	1	2	8	8	8	2		4	4	0.5
Pseudomonas aeruginosa	R	R	R	R	R	R	R	R	R	R	R	R	R	16–R
Bacteroides fragilis	32	32			32	R	R			R		4–32	8–64	0.25

R = minimum inhibitory concentration >32 μg/ml.
Many strains show wide strain variation and considerable inoculum effect.

Reproduced with permission, from Garrod LP, Lambert HP, O'Grady F. In: Antibiotic and Chemotherapy. 5th ed. London: Churchill Livingstone, 1981: 102.

have a broadly similar range of activity, gentamicin being slightly more active against *E. coli* and *Serratia* sp., while tobramycin is more effective against *Pseudomonas aeruginosa* (36). Bacterial resistance can develop against all of the aminoglycosides, mainly induced by plasmid-mediated enzyme production, and cross-resistance between all of the aminoglycosides is common. However, some of the aminoglycosides are immune to the effects of certain of the enzymes and cross-resistance is not universal. Thus netilmicin will often be effective against gram-negative organisms, including *E. coli*, which are resistant to gentamicin and tobramycin (36).

Of the four aminoglycosides under consideration, amikacin has proved to be the most stable, and many gram-negative organisms which are resistant to other aminoglycosides are sensitive to amikacin. In particular, several studies have found little increase in the occurrence of gram-negative resistance to amikacin following its introduction as first-line treatment for suspected sepsis in both adults and children (36); some of these studies have even reported a reduction in the level of resistance to the other aminoglycosides.

Therefore, when both safety and efficacy are taken into account, there are good theoretical reasons for believing that netilmicin is the aminoglycoside of choice for routine use, with a penicillin, for the treatment of suspected sepsis in the newborn, keeping amikacin in reserve for resistant organisms. The netilmicin/penicillin combination has been used in several clinical trials involving the newborn and has been reported to be both safe and effective (4, 38, 39). For those who feel that the side-effects are not a major consideration, assuming that blood levels are monitored adequately, amikacin is an attractive candidate for first-line treatment, in view of its broad spectrum of activity and the apparently low level of resistance associated with its use. There are still many informed and experienced paediatricians, however, who are of the view that gentamicin remains the aminoglycoside of choice in clinical practice.

The cephalosporins

Because of their wide range of activity, the cephalosporins have been used with increasing frequency in the treatment of newborn babies. In view of its activity against most gram-positive, and many gram-negative, organisms, cefuroxime, a second-generation cephalosporin, has been used in some neonatal units; however, the gram-negative cover provided by this antibiotic is limited and probably inadequate for the blind treatment of suspected neonatal sepsis (Table 11.6). These reservations do not apply to many of the third-generation cephalosporins; those which have been studied in the newborn include cefotaxime, ceftazidime and moxalactam.

Reports of the use of cefotaxime in neonates have been generally favourable (4, 40, 41). As with ceftazidime, no serious physical adverse effects have been reported with cefotaxime, which is active against a broad range of organisms. Gram-negative organisms which most frequently cause early neonatal sepsis in this country – *E. coli*, *Klebsiella* sp., *Proteus* sp. and *Haemophilus* sp. – are invariably sensitive to cefotaxime, and the minimum inhibitory concentrations (MICs) for such organisms are often lower than those for the aminoglycosides (5). A further advantage is that cefotaxime shows low MICs against group B streptococci, although there is no synergism with penicillin or ampicillin (42). There have been only isolated reports of the use of cefotaxime in neonatal group B streptococcal sepsis but, to date, there have been no indications that it is less effective than would be predicted by *in-vitro* measurements.

The main disadvantages of cefotaxime are that it is ineffective against *L. monocytogenes* and many *Pseudomonas* spp. and that its use leads to the proliferation of organisms such as *Streptococcus faecalis* and *Enterobacter cloacae*, which are, or may readily become, resistant not only to cefotaxime but also to most other beta-lactam antibiotics. Two neonatal units have reported the emergence of *Ent. cloacae* resistant to the third-generation cephalosporins. In one of these units the resistant organisms appeared following the introduction of cefuroxime as a regular form of treatment for possible infection with *Staph. epidermidis*, and two deaths occurred in babies whose *Ent. cloacae* septicaemia was treated with cefotaxime (2). In four of the infants treated with cefotaxime there was a loss of sensitivity to this antibiotic during the course of treatment; there have been similar reports in adult patients (43). In the other neonatal unit the resistant organisms were detected following the introduction of cefotaxime plus ampicillin as routine first-line treatment for suspected sepsis; although there were six cases of septicaemia, there were no deaths (44). The role of cefotaxime in the treatment of babies who may be infected with organisms with the potential for the production of inducible beta-lactamases, such as *Pseudomonas* sp., *Serratia* sp. and *Enterobacter* sp., is likely, therefore, to be limited. However, this restriction applies largely to babies with suspected *late* sepsis, since these organisms rarely cause early sepsis. In terms of safety and efficacy, cefotaxime alone, or in combination with penicillin or ampicillin for cover against infection with *Listeria*, is an alternative to the combination of an aminoglycoside with penicillin or ampicillin to treat suspected *early* sepsis. However, the implications of such a policy on the subsequent pattern of colonization and late infections require further evaluation.

Ceftazidime has also been evaluated in the treatment of suspected neonatal sepsis (13, 45–48). Like cefotaxime it appears to be safe and there is good penetration into the CSF. The activity of ceftazidime against group B streptococcus is probably not as good as that of cefotaxime and, in the study reported by Low et al., two babies with group B streptococcal sepsis died while being treated with ceftazidime (12). These observations, together with the known poor activity of the third-generation cephalosporins against *L. monocytogenes*, have led to reservations about the use of ceftazidime in the treatment of suspected early sepsis, certainly as monotherapy. The main strength of ceftazidime lies in its gram-negative activity, particularly against *Pseudomonas* sp.; it would seem that ceftazidime is, therefore, more suitable for use in the treatment of late-onset sepsis in which infection with these organisms is suspected or proven.

Moxalactam has also been investigated as a treatment for suspected neonatal sepsis (49) and for neonatal meningitis (50). Although it has useful antimicrobial properties, moxalactam shows poor activity against group B streptococcus; it has been reported to produce a haemorrhagic diathesis in older patients and there is *in-vitro* evidence that it may cause an increase in unbound bilirubin levels (51). Until such doubts about the safety of this antibiotic have been resolved, it is unlikely to have a major role in the routine treatment of neonatal sepsis.

In-vitro studies have indicated that other cephalosporins decrease the reserve albumin concentration in serum in the newborn and may, therefore, be associated with an increased risk of bilirubin encephalopathy. These include ceftriaxone, cefoperazone, cefonicid, cefotetan and cefmetazole (52, 53); however, cefotaxime, ceftazidime and cefuroxime appear to be quite safe in this respect, as do most of the commonly used penicillins (54).

Many of the third-generation cephalosporins have been associated with chromosomally mediated beta-lactamase induction, and an increased prevalence of colonization with *Strep. faecalis* also occurs, the clinical significance of which is not yet clear. However, at least one unit has reported that, because of this increased colonization, ampicillin was added to the treatment regimens of babies receiving ceftazidime for longer than 5 days (13).

Ampicillin

In most neonatal units ampicillin monotherapy can no longer be regarded as appropriate treatment for suspected sepsis, in view of the frequency of resistant coliforms. However, ampicillin is often used in combination with either an aminoglycoside or a cephalosporin, particularly when infection with *L. monocytogenes* is suspected or proven. A recent study from Stockholm reported that an increased rate of carriage of beta-lactam-resistant strains of *E. coli* and *Klebsiella* sp. was found in babies from units in which ampicillin was frequently used; no such association was found with the use of cefuroxime (55). It has been suggested that the potent beta-lactamase-inducing action of ampicillin, combined with the high levels which are usually present in the faeces, predisposes to the proliferation of antibiotic-resistant organisms (56). If such organisms are shown to be the cause of clinical sepsis, these observations could have important implications for the formulation of antibiotic policies in those units in which there is a high incidence of infection caused by *L. monocytogenes*, since ampicillin is currently the treatment of choice for this organism.

Piperacillin

Of the newer penicillins, piperacillin has been the most widely used for the treatment of suspected sepsis in the newborn. The advantages of this antibiotic are that it is safe, when used in older patients, and has good activity against many of the potential neonatal pathogens such as the group B streptococcus and *L. monocytogenes*. In a study which compared piperacillin plus flucloxacillin with gentamicin plus penicillin in the treatment of suspected bacterial infection in infants less than 48 h of age, Placzek et al. found piperacillin to be satisfactory and concluded that it is a safe and effective first-line treatment for early neonatal infection (11). However, some ampicillin-resistant *E. coli* are resistant to piperacillin (16), and piperacillin has poor activity against staphylococci; it is unlikely, therefore, that this antibiotic will be widely used as monotherapy for suspected early sepsis.

Like ceftazidime, piperacillin undoubtedly has an important place in the treatment of specific *Pseudomonas* infections in the neonate. As with other ureidopenicillins, prolongation of the bleeding time has been reported to be associated with the administration of piperacillin in older subjects and this potential disadvantage warrants further investigation (57).

Microbiological surveillance

Recommendations concerning microbiological surveillance vary widely. In 1978 Sprunt et al., on the basis of their study of the development of the pharyngeal flora of neonates in an intensive care unit, recommended that high-risk neonates should have throat swabs taken two to three times per week until a normal pattern is achieved – the normal pattern consisting of the predominance of alpha-haemolytic streptococci (58). In this study nearly all of the organisms which caused infection in the infants, including septicaemia, were present in cultures of oropharyngeal swabs. Similarly, during two outbreaks of serious neonatal infections in Liverpool, one caused by *Klebsiella* (59) and the other by *Ent. cloacae* (2), it was found that the results of routine microbiological surveillance of surface and rectal swabs correlated well with the results of blood and CSF cultures during the outbreak.

In contrast, a surveillance study conducted in the Infant Special Care Unit at the Johns Hopkins Hospital in Baltimore was unable to show that weekly cultures from the nares, umbilicus and rectum were of value in predicting outbreaks of neonatal sepsis caused by gram-negative bacilli, in particular by ampicillin/gentamicin-resistant *Klebsiella* (60). This study also showed no relationship between the frequency of antibiotic usage and rates of either colonization or sepsis with resistant bacteria; similar results were also reported from Oxford (61).

In Oxford it has also been established that the bacteria found in nasopharyngeal and surface swabs (excluding endotracheal secretions) are not necessarily the same as those causing septicaemia in the same infant: in a survey of 26 episodes of late-onset septicaemia the bacteria found in blood cultures corresponded with those found on surface swabs in only 10 cases. Aminoglycoside-resistance patterns in the organisms found on surface swabs did not necessarily occur in the organisms isolated from blood cultures (15).

On the Special Care Baby Unit in Southampton, where cefotaxime has been the main first-line antibiotic used for the past 8 years, routine surveillance cultures are not performed. However, from the results of a recent study in which cefotaxime was compared with netilmicin plus penicillin, it is apparent that many babies, whether they have been treated with cefotaxime or not, become colonized with gram-negative rods which are resistant to cefotaxime (Table 11.7). To date, this has not been associated with outbreaks of clinically proven sepsis, there have been no known deaths from late bacterial sepsis, and no cases of confirmed late gram-negative meningitis have been diagnosed.

A large study of the value of surface cultures in the prediction of true sepsis, which was recently conducted in Nashville, showed that, when cultures were taken from surface sites (ear, nasopharynx, axilla, umbilicus, groin, rectum, stomach and endotracheal tube), their sensitivity, specificity and positive predictive value in predicting invasive infection were only 56%, 82% and 7.5% respectively when taken at the time of suspected sepsis; cultures taken earlier were of even less predictive value (62). Similar findings were reported from Dublin (63). The results of these studies support the view of Klein, who has suggested that routine surveillance cultures, which can be extremely costly, are unnecessary, provided that clinicians have adequate information concerning documented infections and are aware of the local antimicrobial susceptibilities of organisms known to cause disease in neonates (5). For those clinicians who prefer to have some knowledge of the prevailing organisms on their unit, an acceptable compromise may be to undertake less frequent surveillance – perhaps every one or two months.

Table 11.7. *Sensitivity of gram-negative rods to cefotaxime: peripheral isolates (Southampton 1986)*

Day of treatment	No. of isolates sensitive to CTX/no. tested	
	CTX treated	N + P treated
0	16/16 (100%)	14/14 (100%)
2/3	7/11 (64%)	11/11 (100%)
4+	5/13 (38%)	8/13 (62%)

CTX, cefotaxime; N + P, netilmicin plus penicillin.

For ventilated babies, many clinicians feel that routine culture of endotracheal secretions *is* justified and of potential clinical relevance. In Liverpool such secretions were cultured daily (2) and in Oxford weekly (15).

The treatment of suspected late sepsis

As indicated earlier, treatment for episodes of suspected late sepsis probably accounts for a relatively small proportion of the total antibiotic usage on neonatal units. The organisms to be covered in this situation are more wide-ranging than those encountered in early sepsis and almost any antibiotic regimen will leave some possible pathogens uncovered. Bacteria which cause late sepsis include gram-negative bacilli, *Staph. aureus*, *Staph. epidermidis* and *Strep. faecalis*. While anaerobic infections are uncommon (5), the initial clinical signs of late sepsis can be similar to those observed in necrotizing enterocolitis, for which anaerobic cover is usually included (64).

Recommendations for the treatment of suspected late sepsis have included: gentamicin plus penicillin (65), an aminoglycoside plus ampicillin (16), gentamicin plus flucloxacillin (15), and an aminoglycoside plus vancomycin for infants with indwelling vascular catheters (16). Although *Staph. aureus* is still likely to be sensitive to penicillinase-resistant penicillins and, less certainly, to some aminoglycosides, *Staph. epidermidis* is often resistant to most antibiotics except vancomycin. It is generally advised that the blind treatment of suspected late sepsis should take account of the antibiotic sensitivity patterns of recent proven infections occurring in babies in each individual nursery, rather than the patterns found in colonizing organisms (5, 15, 16).

A commonly held view is that the third-generation cephalosporins, particularly ceftazidime, have a place in the treatment of late sepsis at times of outbreaks of infection with aminoglycoside-resistant organisms and, as with piperacillin, in the treatment, often in combination with other agents, of infections of known cause, such as *Pseudomonas*. The antibiotic management of meningitis is discussed in Chapter 9.

Antifungal agents

With the improvement in the survival rates of babies of very low birthweight there has been an increase in the reported incidences of systemic fungal infections among this group of neonates (66). Predisposing factors include extreme prematurity, the use of central venous catheters for parenteral nutrition and the extensive use of broad-spectrum antibiotics. In a recent prospective study Baley et al. reported a fungal colonization rate of 27% for babies of very low birthweight (< 1500 g); of these, 7.7% (2% of the whole group) developed systemic fungal infections (67). The reported mortality rates from neonatal systemic infection are high (68). It is possible also that, as in older patients whose immunity is compromised, fungal colonization of areas of the upper digestive tract, such as the oesophagus, may provide portals of entry for bacteria. The treatment and prophylaxis of neonate fungal infections are, therefore, subjects of increasing interest to those involved in the care of the newborn.

The administration of prophylactic nystatin is now commonplace in many neonatal units (69, 70), although the efficacy of such a policy is still unclear. Of the five neonates with systemic fungal infections reported by Johnson et al., four had received prophylactic oral nystatin before developing the systemic disease (68); however, all of these infants survived. The first randomized controlled trial of nystatin prophylaxis in infants weighing less than 1250 g at birth has recently been reported (71). Fungal colonization and infection rates were found to be lower in the babies receiving prophylactic nystatin, and mortality was higher in the babies who were colonized with fungi; however, the number of babies in the control group who developed systemic fungal sepsis was much higher (32%) than in other studies. Further controlled trials, in larger populations of patients, are needed to evaluate the efficacy of prophylactic antifungal therapy in neonates.

The results of studies of older patients at risk of developing fungal infections have been mixed (72, 73). With nystatin prophylaxis the emergence of resistant strains has been extremely uncommon, but this may not be the case with amphotericin B (73). There is no information available concerning the prophylactic use in the newborn of amphotericin B, the other main polyene antifungal agent or ketoconazole, and imidazole-dioxolane. Since ketoconazole is systemically absorbed after oral administration and hepatotoxicity has been reported, there must be reservations about its use as a prophylactic agent in preterm infants. Thus, as an operational policy, the routine use of nystatin can be advocated, since it is known to be safe in older patients and does not significantly promote the development of resistant organisms; its efficacy in preventing either local or invasive fungal infection, however, is not proven.

For established systemic fungal infections the current treatment of choice for the neonate is probably a combination of amphotericin B and 5-flucytosine (68); Smith and Congdon have suggested that 5-flucytosine alone may be adequate for babies who do not have fulminating illness or multi-organ involvement (70). There is no consensus on the duration of treatment, but Smith and Congdon have recommended treating for 10–14 days initially and using urine cultures as a means of assessing the need for treatment thereafter. As with the aminoglycosides, although these agents are known to have significant side-effects in older children and adults, they have been well tolerated in neonates (68).

Future approaches to infection in the neonate

While the search for safer and more effective antibiotics continues unabated, there is also increasing interest in exploring different methods of controlling bacterial and fungal infections in the newborn. Two of these will be considered in more detail here.

Colonization resistance

The concept of colonization resistance has held currency for many years, much of the original work being concerned with the microbiological effects of irradiation of laboratory animals (74). In essence, the concept is based on the theory that, if the anaerobic flora of the bowel is preserved and promoted, it can prevent subsequent colonization with, and hence invasion by, pathogenic organisms. There is some evidence from work with laboratory animals to support this contention and the concept has been used, with variable success, in the management of patients receiving chemotherapy (75). More recently, the idea has been applied to the management of patients with normal immune mechanisms who are receiving intensive care. Such patients are at risk of becoming infected with hospital-acquired organisms.

In order to preserve and promote a favourable anaerobic flora, the patients are treated with a cocktail of orally administered, non-absorbed antibiotics – tobramycin, polymixin E and amphotericin B – while receiving a broad-spectrum antibiotic such as cefotaxime parenterally to prevent systemic infection by organisms originating primarily from the respiratory tract (76). The aim of this therapy is to eliminate the potentially pathogenic aerobic flora from the digestive tract, while maintaining the beneficial anaerobic organisms, thus achieving 'selective digestive decontamination'. Preliminary trials have indicated a remarkable reduction in the rate of hospital-acquired infections (77). However, it is not yet clear whether there is a concomitant reduction in the mortality rate of patients treated by this method. There are also theoretical concerns that the widespread use of antibiotics in this way may lead to the emergence of pathogenic organisms which are resistant to most, if not all, antibiotics.

There have been no reports of the application of the technique of selective digestive decontamination to patients on neonatal intensive care units. It is possible that the technique, or appropriate modifications, could be applied in the newborn period since, unlike adults, neonates have no existing aerobic flora to impede the establishment of the anaerobic flora. It is likely, however, that different, and possibly safer, antibiotic agents would be required for use in neonates, since those used in the studies on adult patients may be absorbed from the digestive tract of newborn infants.

Probiotics

Before concluding this chapter it would be appropriate to consider the concept of *probiotics*. Probiosis is defined as 'a mutual association of two organisms that benefits or enhançes the life processes of both' (78). In recent years the notion of administering probiotics, rather than antibiotics, has excited some attention in the field of animal husbandry, the aim being to encourage the development of the type of gastrointestinal bacterial flora in livestock which is beneficial for the growth and wellbeing of animals which are reared for commercial purposes. Since some of the organisms which cause sepsis in neonates originate from an abnormally colonized bowel, the idea of administering probiotics – bacteria which are of benefit to the host – is worthy of consideration and is, perhaps, a natural progression from the concept of selective digestive decontamination (79).

One of the problems encountered in attempting to induce a favourable intestinal bacterial flora in the newborn is that there are difficulties in defining the normal bowel flora of normal neonates (80). While earlier studies indicated that the stool of the normal full-term breast-fed infant is different from that of bottle-fed babies and is predominantly characterized by the presence of bifidobacteria and relatively few coliform bacteria (81), more recent work has indicated that the stool flora of bottle-fed babies is similar to that of breast-fed infants (82, 83). There is also some evidence to suggest that the stool bacterial content of babies from industrialized countries is different from that found in babies from pre-industrialized societies (84).

There have been two recent studies in which live bacteria were administered to newborn infants. In the first, conducted by Sprunt et al., the aim was not to influence the colonization of the bowel, but to induce a 'normal' flora (alpha-haemolytic streptococci) in the nasopharynx (85). In an uncontrolled study 22 newborn infants in a neonatal intensive care unit received a single nasopharyngeal implantation of a strain of alpha-haemolytic streptococci. In 16 of these infants the implant strain was found to constitute the predominant nasopharyngeal flora within 48–72 h of implantation. It is not clear whether this conferred any advantage on these infants and any follow-up controlled trials which may have been undertaken do not appear to have been published.

More recently, Reuman et al., in a controlled trial, administered live *Lactobacillus acidophilus* to 15 premature infants within 72 h of delivery (86). Although they were able to show a significant difference in the rates of lactobacillus colonization between the study and the control patients, they found no difference between the two groups in the number of gram-negative organisms present in the stool or in the number of aminoglycoside-resistant gram-negative organisms. They were unable also to show any statistically significant difference in morbidity or mortality between the study groups. Other types of lactobacilli and bifidobacteria are currently under investigation for their suitability for use as probiotics in the newborn period (79).

Acknowledgements

I thank Dr Andrew Lowes, Director of the Southampton PHLS for his invaluable advice and Dr Tony Ducker, Consultant Paediatrician at All Saints' Hospital, Chatham, for his permission to include the data concerning his patients.

References

1. Silverman WA. Retrolental fibroplasia: a modern parable. New York: Grune and Stratton, 1980: 79-82.
2. Modi N, Damjanovic V, Cooke RWI. Outbreak of cephalosporin resistant *Enterobacter cloacae* infection in a neonatal intensive care unit. Arch Dis Child 1987; 62: 148-51.
3. Hammerschlag MR, Klein JO, Herschel M, Chen FCJ, Fermin R. Patterns of use of antibiotics in two newborn nurseries. N Engl J Med 1977; 296: 1268-9.
4. Hall MA, Ducker DA, Lowes JA et al. A randomised prospective comparison of cefotaxime versus netilmicin/penicillin for treatment of suspected neonatal sepsis. Drugs 1988; 35(suppl 2): 169-77.
5. Klein JO. Infectious diseases in the newborn infant. Adv Pediatr 1984; 31: 405-46.
6. Forfar JO. Neonatal infection. In: Forfar JO, Arneil GC (eds) Textbook of paediatrics. 3rd ed. Edinburgh: Churchill Livingstone, 1984: 204-7.
7. Placzek MM, Whitelaw A. Early and late neonatal septicaemia. Arch Dis Child 1983; 58: 728-31.
8. Vesikari T, Janas M, Gronroos P et al. Neonatal septicaemia. Arch Dis Child 1985; 60: 542-6.
9. Hensey OJ, Hart CA, Cooke RWI. Serious infection in a neonatal intensive care unit: a two-year survey. J Hyg Camb 1985; 95: 289-97.
10. Baker CJ. Group B streptococcal infections. Adv Int Med 1980; 25: 475-501.
11. Placzek M, Whitelaw A, Want S, Sahathevan M, Darrell J. Piperacillin in early neonatal infection. Arch Dis Child 1983; 58: 1006-9.
12. Low DC, Bissenden JG, Wise R. Ceftazidime in neonatal infection. Arch Dis Child 1985; 60: 360-4.
13. Mulhall A, de Louvois J. Two years experience with ceftazidime in neonatal practice. In: Duerden BI, Caldwell D (eds) Antibiotic therapy in at-risk neonates: the place of ceftazidime. (Insights into the treatment of serious infections, vol 1.) Macclesfield: Gardiner-Caldwell Communications, 1985: 167-73.
14. Philip AGS, Hewitt JR. Early diagnosis of neonatal sepsis. Pediatrics 1980; 65: 1036-41.
15. Isaacs D, Wilkinson AR. Antibiotic use in the neonatal unit. Arch Dis Child 1987; 62: 204-8.
16. Starr SE. Antimicrobial therapy of bacterial sepsis in the newborn infant. J Pediatr 1985; 106: 1043-8.
17. Editorial. Deafness in low birthweight infants: is it avoidable? Lancet 1985; 1: 1373-4.
18. Hauch A-M, Peitersen B, Peitersen E. Vestibular toxicity following netilmicin therapy in the neonatal period. Dan Med Bull 1986; 33: 107-9.
19. McCracken GH. Aminoglycoside toxicity in infants and children. Am J Med 1986; 80 (suppl 6B): 172-8.
20. Finitzo-Hieber T, McCracken GH, Brown KC. Prospective controlled evaluation of auditory function in neonates given netilmicin or amikacin. J Pediatr 1985; 106: 129-36.
21. Davey P. Aminoglycosides and neonatal deafness. Lancet 1985; 1: 612.
22. Rajchgot P, Prober CG, Soldin S et al. Aminoglycoside-related nephrotoxicity in the premature newborn. Clin Pharmacol Ther 1984; 35: 394-401.
23. Giacoia GP, Schentag JJ. Pharmacokinetics and nephrotoxicity of continuous intravenous infusion of gentamicin in low birth weight infants. J Pediatr 1986; 109: 715-19.
24. Tessin I, Bergmark J, Hiesche K, Jagenburg R, Trollfors B. Renal function of neonates during gentamicin treatment. Arch Dis Child 1982; 57: 758-60.
25. Adelman RD, Wirth F, Rubio T. A controlled study of the nephrotoxicity of mezlocillin and gentamicin plus ampicillin in the neonate. J Pediatr 1987; 111: 888-93.
26. Tilstone WJ, Semple PF, Lawson DH, Boyle JA. Effects of furosemide on glomerular filtration rate and clearance of practolol, digoxin, cephaloridine and gentamicin. Clin Pharmacol Ther 1977; 22: 389-94.
27. Zarfin Y, Koren G, Maresky D, Perlman M, MacLeod S. Possible indomethacin-aminoglycoside interaction in preterm infants. J Pediatr 1985; 106: 511-13.
28. Keller H, Bircher J. Miscellaneous antibiotics. In: Dukes MNG (ed) Meyler's side effects of drugs. 9th ed. Amsterdam: Excerpta Medica, 1980: 457.

29. Santos JI, Swenson P, Glasgow L. Potentiation of *Clostridium botulinum* toxin by aminoglycoside antibiotics. Pediatrics 1981; 68: 50–4.
30. L'Hommedieu CS, Nicholas D, Armes DA, Jones P, Nelson T, Pickering LK. Potentiation of magnesium sulfate-induced neuromuscular weakness by gentamicin, tobramycin and amikacin. J Pediatr 1983; 102: 629–31.
31. Klein JO. Antimicrobial agents for infants and children. In: Feigin RD, Cherry JD (eds) Textbook of pediatric infectious diseases. Philadelphia: WB Saunders, 1981: 1702.
32. Stutman HR, Marks MI. Therapy for bacterial meningitis: which drugs, and for how long? J Pediatr 1987; 110: 812–14.
33. Milner RDG, Ross J, Froud DJR, Davis JA. Clinical pharmacology of gentamicin in the newborn infant. Arch Dis Child 1972; 47: 927–32.
34. Milner RDG. Netilmicin in the newborn. In: Richardson RG (ed Netilmicin: a recent advance in aminoglycoside therapy. Royal Society of Medicine International Congress and Symposium Series No. 50. London: Academic Press and Royal Society of Medicine, 1982: 157–61.
35. Kahlmeter G, Dahlager JI. Aminoglycoside toxicity: a review of clinical studies published between 1975 and 1982. J Antimicrob Chemother 1984; 13(suppl A): 9–22.
36. Siegenthaler WE, Bonetti A, Luthy R. Aminoglycoside antibiotics in infectious diseases. Am J Med 1986; 80(suppl 6B): 2–14.
37. Lerner AM, Reyes MP, Cone LA, Blair DC, Jansen W, Wright GE, Lorber RR. Randomised, controlled trial of the comparative efficacy, auditory toxicity, and nephrotoxicity of tobramycin and netilmicin. Lancet 1983; 1: 1123–6.
38. Michalsen H, Halvorsen K, Bergan T. Netilmicin in the treatment of neonates with moderate and severe infections. Scand J Infect Dis 1980; 23: 146–50.
39. Trujillo H, Manotas R, Loaiza J. Safety and efficacy of netilmicin in neonates with serious systemic infections. J Int Med Res 1981; 9: 52–7.
40. de Louvois J, Mulhall A, Hurley R. The safety and pharmacokinetics of cefotaxime in the treatment of neonates. Pediatr Pharmacol 1982; 2: 275–84.
41. Hall MA, Beech RC, Seal DV. The use of cefotaxime for treating suspected neonatal sepsis: 2 years' experience. J Hosp Infect 1986; 8: 57–63.
42. Landesman SH, Corrado ML, Cherubin CE, Sierra MF. Activity of moxalactam and cefotaxime alone and in combination with ampicillin or penicillin against group B streptococci. Antimicrob Agents Chemother 1981; 19: 794–7.
43. Svarva PL, Lyng RV, Maeland JA. Emergence of beta-lactam multiresistant variants of gram-negative bacilli in the presence of cefotaxime. Scand J Infect Dis 1985; 17: 387–91.
44. Bryan CS, John JF, Pai S, Austin TL. Gentamicin vs. cefotaxime for therapy of neonatal sepsis. Am J Dis Child 1985; 139: 1086–9.
45. Snelling S, Hart CA, Cooke RWI. Ceftazidime or gentamicin plus benzylpenicillin in neonates less than 48 hours old. J Antimicrob Chemother 1983; 12(suppl A): 353–6.
46. Pollock I, Mulhall A, de Louvois J. Ceftazidime in the treatment of neonatal infection. J Hosp Infect 1985; 6: 158–65.
47. Arimasu O, Hashira S, Fujii R. Clinical evaluation of ceftazidime in the treatment of neonatal infection. Jpn J Antibiot 1986; 39: 2077–83.
48. Elias-Jones AC. A randomised comparative study of ceftazidime versus gentamicin plus benzylpenicillin in neonates with signs of serious infections. Insights Treat Serious Infect 1985; 1: 191–7.
49. de Louvois J, James J, Mulhall A. Latamoxef and the newborn. Arch Dis Child 1984; 59: 346–50.
50. McCracken GH Jr, Threlkeld N, Mize S et al. Moxalactam therapy for neonatal meningitis due to gram-negative enteric bacilli. J Am Med Assoc 1984; 252: 1427–32.
51. Stutman HR, Parker KM, Marks MI. Potential of moxalactam and other new antimicrobial agents for bilirubin–albumin displacement in neonates. Pediatrics 1985; 75: 294–8.
52. Fink S, Karp W, Robertson A. Ceftriaxone effect on bilirubin–albumin binding. Pediatrics 1987; 80: 873–5.
53. Robertson A, Fink S, Karp W. Effect of cephalosporins on bilirubin–albumin binding. J Pediatr 1988; 112: 291–4.
54. Fink S, Karp W, Robertson A. Effect of penicillins on bilirubin–albumin binding. J Pediatr 1988; 113: 566–8.
55. Tullus K, Burman LG. Ecological impact of ampicillin and cefuroxime in neonatal units. Lancet 1989; 1: 1405–7.
56. van Saene R, Leonard M, Shears P. Ecological impact of antibiotics in neonatal units. Lancet 1989; 2: 509–10.

57. Lee M, Stobnicki M, Sharifi R. Haemorrhagic complications of piperacillin therapy. J Urol 1986; 136: 454–5.
58. Sprunt K, Leidy G, Redman W. Abnormal colonization of neonates in an intensive care unit: means of identifying neonates at risk of infection. Pediatr Res 1978; 12: 998–1002.
59. Morgan MEI, Hart CA, Cooke RWI. Klebsiella infection in a neonatal intensive care unit: role of bacteriological surveillance. J Hosp Infect 1984; 5: 377–85.
60. White RD, Townsend TR, Stephens MA, Moxon ER. Are surveillance of resistant enteric bacilli and antimicrobial usage among neonates in a newborn intensive care unit useful? Pediatrics 1981; 68: 1–4.
61. Isaacs D, Catterson J, Hope PL, Moxon ER, Wilkinson AR. Factors influencing colonisation with gentamicin resistant gram negative organisms in the neonatal unit. Arch Dis Child 1988; 63: 533–5.
62. Evans ME, Schaffner W, Federspiel CF, Cotton RB, McKee KT Jr, Stratton CW. Sensitivity, specificity and predictive value of body surface cultures in a neonatal intensive care unit. J Am Med Assoc 1988; 259: 248–52.
63. Fox GP, Clarke TA, Matthews TG. Are routine superficial cultures worthwhile in neonatal practice? Br Med J 1988; 296: 1443.
64. Hall P, Kaye CM, McIntosh N, Steele J. Intravenous metronidazole in the newborn. Arch Dis Child 1983; 58: 529–31.
65. Siegel JD, McCracken GH Jr. Sepsis neonatorum. N Engl J Med 1981; 304: 642–47.
66. Knox WF, Hooton VN, Barson AJ. Pulmonary vascular candidiasis and use of central venous catheters in neonates. J Clin Pathol 1987; 40: 559–65.
67. Baley JE, Kliegman RM, Boxerbaum B, Fanaroff AA. Fungal colonization in the very low birth weight infant. Pediatrics 1986; 78: 225–32.
68. Johnson DE, Thompson TR, Green TP, Ferrieri P. Systemic candidiasis in very low-birth-weight infants (< 1500 grams). Pediatrics 1984; 73: 138–43.
69. Pearse RG, Roberton NRC. Infection in the neonate. In: Roberton NRC (ed) Textbook of neonatology. Edinburgh: Churchill Livingstone, 1976: 776.
70. Smith H, Congdon P. Neonatal systemic candidiasis. Arch Dis Child 1985; 60: 365–9.
71. Sims ME, Yoo Y, You H, Salminen C, Walther FJ. Prophylactic oral nystatin and fungal infections in very-low-birthweight infants. Am J Perinatol 1988; 5: 33–6.
72. Meunier-Carpentier F. Chemoprophylaxis of fungal infections. Am J Med 1984; 76: 652–6.
73. Meunier F. Prevention of mycoses in immunocompromised patients. Rev Infect Dis 1987; 9: 408–15.
74. van der Waaij D. The persistent absence of Enterobacteriaceae from the intestinal flora of mice following antibiotic treatment. J Infect Dis 1968; 118: 32–8.
75. Schimpff SC. Infection prevention in patients with cancer and granulocytopenia. In: Greco MH (ed) Infections in the abnormal host. New York: Yorke, 1980: 935–49.
76. Stoutenbeek CP, van Saene HKF, Miranda DR, Zandstra DF, Binnendijk B. The prevention of superinfection in multiple trauma patients. J Antimicrob Chemother 1984; 14 (suppl B): 203–11.
77. Ledingham IM, Alcock SR, Eastaway AT, McDonald JC, McKay IC, Ramsay G. Triple regimen of selective decontamination of the digestive tract, systemic cefotaxime, and microbiological surveillance for prevention of acquired infection in intensive care. Lancet 1988; 1: 785–90.
78. Becker EL, Landau SI (eds). International dictionary of medicine and biology, vol III. New York: Wiley, 1986: 2296.
79. Goldmann DA. The bacterial flora of neonates in intensive care: monitoring and manipulation. J Hosp Infect 1988; 11 (suppl A): 340–51.
80. Rolles CJ, Hall MA, Duncan H, Sampeys C. Bifidobacteria and breast milk: a review and an hypothesis. In: Wharton B (ed) Tropics in perinatal medicine, vol 2. London: Pitman, 1982: 31–47.
81. Bullen CL, Tearle PV, Stewart MG. The effect of 'humanised' milks and supplemented breast feeding on the faecal flora of infants. J Med Microbiol 1977; 10: 403–13.
82. Yoshioka H, Isaki K, Fujita K. Development and differences of intestinal flora in the neonatal period in breast-fed and bottle-fed infants. Pediatrics 1983; 72: 317–21.
83. Hall MA, Cole CB, Smith S, Fuller R, Rolles CJ. Factors influencing the presence of faecal lactobacilli in early infancy. Arch Dis Child (in press).

84. Simhon A, Douglas JR, Draser BS, Soothill JF. Effect of feeding on infants' faecal flora. Arch Dis Child 1982; 57: 54–8.
85. Sprunt K, Leidy G, Redman W. Abnormal colonization of neonates in an ICU: conversion to normal colonization by pharyngeal implantation of alpha hemolytic streptococcus strain 215. Pediatr Res 1980; 14: 308–13.
86. Reuman PD, Duckworth DH, Smith KL, Kagan R. Bucciarelli RL, Ayoub EM. Lack of effect of *Lactobacillus* on gastro-intestinal bacterial colonisation in premature infants. Pediatr Infect Dis 1986; 5: 663–8.

12 Infection in the Mother

A. B. MacLean
University of Glasgow, UK

The problem of infection in the newborn cannot be considered without regard to the mother. This chapter describes infection in the pregnant woman, the means by which the fetus is exposed to infecting organisms, and how infection is transmitted at birth.

Maternal infection

There is little dispute that some infections show different clinical patterns and some have more serious sequelae during pregnancy.

Monilial vulvovaginitis

Vulvovaginitis is the most common infection seen in pregnancy. *Candida albicans* is identified in approximately 20% of women seen in antenatal clinics (1). This prevalence is probably no different from that in non-pregnant sexually active women, particularly if these women use combined oral contraceptives. However, during pregnancy there is a greater chance that *Candida* will proliferate and will cause symptomatic infection. This increase is due to altered cervical secretions which produce a rise in pH, and to the frequent occurrence of glycosuria starting even in the first trimester. Apart from discomfort, this infection does not cause other problems for the pregnant mother, and the management is topical application of a fungicide. The risk to the fetus is minimal; the newborn infant is readily colonized, but only the preterm baby receiving intensive care is ever seriously infected by *Candida*.

Bacteriuria

The presence of significant bacteria in the urinary tract is seen in approximately 5% of sexually active women in the UK or USA. The prevalence is increased in some ethnic groups. Pregnancy does not alter the prevalence of bacteriuria, but there is an increased risk of progression to pyelonephritis. This is due to ureteric dilatation from the smooth-muscle effect of progestogens and pressure from an enlarging uterus. It has been known for a long time that pyelonephritis is associated with preterm delivery (2). This can be reduced by screening every pregnant woman for evidence of bacteriuria, treating with appropriate antibiotics, and following up those with identified infection.

Acute peritonitis

Acute appendicitis is the commonest extra-uterine complication of pregnancy requiring laparotomy. Rapid progress to peritonitis is more likely during pregnancy because of delays in making the diagnosis due to poor localization of pain with the ascending position of the appendix and the increased distance between the appendix and abdominal wall. Another reason is the intervention of the

Infection in the Newborn. Edited by J. de Louvois and D. Harvey
©1990 John Wiley & Sons Ltd

gravid uterus, reducing the effect of the omentum. The diagnosis may also be confused with acute pyelonephritis, extrauterine pregnancy, accidents to ovarian cysts including the corpus luteum, acute cholecystitis, acute pancreatitis and other less common intra-abdominal pathologies found during pregnancy. Optimal management requires early surgery and drainage, if necessary, and antibiotics against aerobic and anaerobic gut organisms.

Viral influenza

There is no evidence that pregnant women succumb to the common cold or influenza more frequently than non-pregnant women. However, the sequelae of infection are more serious during pregnancy. This statement is based on the report, published in 1919, of a survey of 1350 cases of influenza contracted during pregnancy (3). Pneumonia complicated the infection in half these patients, and approximately half of those with pneumonia died. Mortality appeared to be greater in the last 3 months of pregnancy. There is little doubt that many of these women had superimposed bacterial infection, which nowadays would be treated with appropriate antibiotics. It is not necessary to vaccinate pregnant women against influenza.

Hepatitis

It appears that non-A, non-B hepatitis during pregnancy is more likely to be fulminant and is associated with high mortality. During the Bombay epidemic the incidence of hepatitis was significantly increased in pregnant women compared to that in non-pregnant women and in men, and the increase was greatest in late pregnancy (4). Furthermore, the hepatitis seen in pregnancy was more likely to be associated with hepatic failure and this risk also increased as pregnancy progressed. The course of hepatitis B is not usually affected by pregnancy.

Varicella

Infection with varicella zoster virus (VZV) is associated with severe pneumonia and sometimes fatal dissemination during pregnancy. Pneumonia was found in four of 43 pregnant women with chicken pox in one study, and one of these died (5). More recently J. C. P. Kingdom (personal communication) has reviewed 31 cases of varicella seen in Glasgow between 1984 and 1989. Over half the patients admitted to hospital with varicella had cough and tachypnoea associated with their rash. Ten women had evidence of lung involvement, four patients required transfer to an intensive care unit, and three required ventilation; one died and one suffered a tracheo-oesophageal fistula secondary to tracheostomy. Severity of respiratory problems correlated with smoking habits and with the delay between seeing the patient with her rash and referring for treatment (with acyclovir).

Listeriosis

Infection with *Listeria monocytogenes* during pregnancy may vary from a trivial or flu-like illness to more serious meningo-encephalitis. The susceptability of pregnant women is not clear, but appears to include a special affinity of the organism for the decidua and the placenta, together with a compromise in cell-mediated immunity. *Listeria* bacteria are frequently carried in the gastrointestinal tract of pregnant women (up to 16%), but carriage is not affected by pregnancy and the outcome of pregnancy is not affected by intestinal carriage. It was previously believed that pregnant women were infected through contact with animals, but recent evidence suggests that infection occurs after the consumption of certain foods including coleslaw, pâté, margarine, soft cheese and other milk products. There is evidence to show that many *Listeria* organisms are of low virulence, but in some circumstances this can change to produce pathogenic strains. Further information on listeriosis is provided in Chapter 5.

Tuberculosis

Tuberculosis during pregnancy is now rare in the developed countries. Some of the complications, such as tuberculous meningitis, may be life-threatening (6). Such problems are often serious because of the delay in diagnosis which may occur because of the non-specific features of the infection and because doctors are insufficiently aware that tuberculosis still occurs. On the other hand, pulmonary tuberculosis is not affected by pregnancy, providing treatment is not stopped.

Malaria

The morbidity and mortality from malaria are higher in pregnant than in non-pregnant women. Pregnancy increases malarial parasitaemia and also increases the incidence of clinical manifestations. *Plasmodium falciparum* may produce acute renal failure in pregnancy, cerebral malaria with coma and convulsions similar to eclampsia. These differences, compared to non-pregnant women, relate to increased cortisol levels in patients with clinical malaria (7). It is uncertain whether this is the reason for the more serious manifestations of malaria in pregnancy or its effect. Although there is concern about teratogenicity associated with malaria chemoprophylaxis, the risks of malaria in pregnancy are too great to stop medication. It is better that pregnant travellers avoid endemic areas.

Amoebic dysentery

This deteriorates during pregnancy, and new infection is likely to produce rapid or fatal progression; latent infection may be reactivated. Occasionally, other intestinal infestations, such as with helminths, may result in a serious increase in parasite burden during pregnancy.

Genital condylomata

It is known that condylomata due to human papillomavirus (HPV), frequently increase in size during pregnancy and undergo regression in the puerperium. It is unknown why HPV produces such epithelial proliferation during pregnancy but, as it is also seen in some patients using combined oral contraceptives, there may be some hormonal basis to this phenomenon. Currently there is uncertainty as to the need to treat condylomata if they are recognized during pregnancy.

Acquired immune deficiency syndrome

Uncertainty exists as to the effect of pregnancy on human immunodeficiency virus (HIV) infection and its progression to a symptomatic disease state. Earlier North American reports suggested that pregnancy was one of the factors associated with disease progression. HIV-positive women were identified because their infants developed acquired immune deficiency syndrome (AIDS) and this was more likely to be associated with antigenaemia during pregnancy. These observations led to the recommendation that pregnant women infected by HIV should be considered for and counselled about termination of pregnancy (8). The Edinburgh data (9) showed no difference in clinical category between those who had a pregnancy following seroconversion and those who did not. Laboratory data showed that the pregnancy group had higher T-helper lymphocyte counts, perhaps because they were less likely to be still using drugs, and thus might be expected to have a better prognosis (see Chapter 8).

Does pregnancy increase risk of maternal infection?

The means by which the mother tolerates her fetal homograft without apparent rejection continues to elude our understanding. The earlier hypothesis that pregnancy is a state of immunosuppression is no longer credible. The Rhesus-negative women will produce antibodies if challenged with Rhesus D antigen during her pregnancy. If exposed to rubella or other viral infection, a pregnant woman will still produce immunoglobulins, thus enabling the diagnosis to be confirmed and the risk of embryopathy suspected. The pregnant renal transplant patient still requires continuing treatment with prednisolone and azathioprine or cyclosporin and will reject the kidney graft during pregnancy if mismanaged.

Nevertheless, there are clinical observations that suggest a degree of immune suppression. Some patients with psoriasis, asthma, or with autoimmune disorders such as systemic lupus erythematosus or rheumatoid arthritis, will improve during pregnancy. The laboratory data on immune changes seen during pregnancy are conflicting. Some of this conflict will arise because changes demonstrated *in vitro* will not necessarily reflect *in-vivo* phenomena. Jones et al. (10) used delayed hypersensitivity skin testing to demonstrate *in-vivo* responses, but found no difference between pregnant and non-pregnant women. They also used a range of *in-vitro* tests and, in some pregnant women, demonstrated enhanced rather than suppressed cell-mediated immunity. However, it is likely that response to viral infection and infections such as listeriosis will depend on cell-mediated immunity with complex interaction between oestrogens, progesterones, prostaglandins, circulating fetoproteins, interleukins and interferons, plus the helper, cytotoxic and suppressor subsets of T lymphocytes, antigen-presenting cells, macrophages and natural killer cells. Recent information (11) suggests that natural killer cells are important in response against the herpes viral infections including VZV and cytomegalovirus. Serum from pregnant women can suppress natural killer cell activity (12). There is a reduction in T-helper lymphocytes during pregnancy, with a return to normal levels by the third to fifth month *post partum* (13). This reduction is greatest in the third trimester. It is also known that immunoglobulins are reduced during pregnancy, but this reduction parallels the fall in serum albumin and may be due to haemodilution (14).

Hopefully, the availability of monoclonal antibodies and more sophisticated tests to define T-lymphocyte and natural killer cell function will possibly enable clarification of the changes in cell immunity seen during pregnancy. There is no doubt that the majority of women no longer face serious infection during pregnancy. However, for a few women in British obstetric practice and for those in developing countries, maternal infection during pregnancy still poses a serious threat.

Transmission of infection to the fetus

The concept that the fetus is in a protected environment *in utero* is outdated. The fetus may be exposed to infection under the following circumstances.

Haematogenous spread

Organisms may reach the fetus across the placenta from the maternal circulation. The presence of organisms in the maternal blood may be associated with signs and symptoms, as in influenza or pyelonephritis, but many episodes will be asymptomatic or associated with trivial maternal illness, such as rash or lymphadenopathy. Some organisms may cross the ‘placental barrier’ without leaving a hint of infection, while others will cause placentitis, with a variety of histopathological changes (15). The organisms which invade in this way include bacteria (gram-negative bacilli and gram-positive cocci, plus *Listeria*, *Treponema* and *Mycobacterium* spp.) protozoa (*Toxoplasma* and *Plasmodium* spp.) and many viruses.

Ascending infection

Organisms may reach the fetus by ascending the vagina and endocervix and infecting the membranes, ruptured or intact, causing chorioamnionitis. The amniotic fluid may be contaminated and then swallowed by the fetus, or infection may spread along the membranes to reach the fetus via the cord, giving rise to funisitis.

The diagnosis of chorioamnionitis is based on the histological demonstration of a polymorph leucocyte infiltration of the membranes, placenta or cord, and the presence of organisms. These may be demonstrated by microscopy (e.g. Gram staining for bacteria or fungi) or by appropriate culture. The clinical features of chorioamnionitis may be minimal, but can include uterine irritability or tenderness, maternal pyrexia, fetal tachycardia, and foul-smelling or discoloured liquor. A review of the literature (15) showed that the incidence of chorioamnionitis varied between 5 and 50% of placentas, and the prevalence of cord infection was between 2 and 39%. *Gardnerella vaginalis*, group B streptococci, *Mycoplasma hominis*, *Ureaplasma urealyticum* and *Candida* spp. are frequently found in the genital tract during pregnancy, but whether they cause chorioamnionitis is still debated (16–18). The integrity of the membranes, cervical immunoglobulins and various anti-bacterial factors (possibly zinc and dietary-related) and lysozymes in the liquor provide some limited protection to the fetus from ascending infection.

Spread associated with fetal investigation

Infection has been found following chorion villus sampling (especially if performed by the transcervical route (19)), amniocentesis, fetoscopy, fetal blood sampling and intra-uterine transfusion. Often the organisms belong to the normal flora of the skin (20) or genital tract, and such cases demonstrate the need not only for skill but also for meticulous aseptic technique during investigative procedures.

Spread from the endometrium

Infection may threaten the fetus in the presence of endometritis and an intrauterine contraceptive device (IUCD). The risk of abortion is greater if an IUCD is left *in utero* than it is with the removal of the device (21). The risk of infection appears to be related to whether the thread protrudes through the cervix, and to the size of the device (as with the Dalkon Shield). The presence of an IUCD in the membranes or placenta does not always cause infection or sequelae and, if the thread is not visible, the pregnancy need not be interrupted.

The effects of fetal infection depend on the organism and the gestation, and may be: nothing; abortion; congenital abnormality; intrauterine death; intrauterine growth retardation; onset of labour; or neonatal sepsis (see Table 12.1).

Infection and abortion

The causes of abortion are numerous and sometimes multiple. The role of infection is confused by the presence of organisms which contaminate the abortus during expulsion, and by inflammatory cells demonstrated histologically in the curettings (22).

Table 12.1. *Effects of infection on the fetus*

Organism	Effect				
	Congenital abnormality	IUD	IUGR	Preterm delivery	Intrapartum transmission to neonate
Viruses					
Cytomegalovirus	Yes	Yes	Yes	No	No
Rubella	Yes	Yes	Yes	?	No
Varicella	Yes	Rare	Yes	Yes	Yes
Herpes simplex	Rare	Rare	?	?	Yes
Influenza	?	Yes	No	Yes	Yes
Coxsackie	No	Yes	Yes	No	Yes
Polio and enterovirus	No	Yes	No	Yes	Yes
Measles	No	Yes	No	?	No
Mumps	? Cardiac	No	No	No	No
Parvo	Unlikely	Yes	No	No	No
Hepatitis B	No	Rare	No	Yes	Yes
Papilloma	No	No	No	?	Rare
Human immuno-deficiency virus	?	No	?	No	Yes
Bacteria					
Treponema	Yes	Yes	Yes	Yes	Yes
Listeria	No	Yes	No	Yes	Yes
Mycoplasma	No	No	Yes	Yes	Yes
Chlamydia	No	No	?	Yes	Yes
Group B streptococci	No	No	No	?	Yes
Protozoa					
Toxoplasma gondii	Yes	Yes	Yes	Yes	Yes
Plasmodium spp.	No	Yes	Yes	Yes	Yes

IUD, intrauterine death; IUGR, intrauterine growth retardation.

Yes, reported evidence; No, no reported evidence; ?, uncertain or conflicting evidence; Rare, reported evidence, but uncommon effect.

Table 12.2 lists organisms that have been associated with spontaneous abortion. Earlier North American claims that *Chlamydia trachomatis*, *M. hominis* and *U. urealyticum* are causes of abortion have been challenged by the findings of recent European studies (22–24). The table includes a number of organisms causing zoonotic infections contracted either via direct contact with animals or by contaminated animal products or food. Although these organisms are well-documented causes of abortion in cattle, pigs, sheep and goats, their role in human abortion is likely to be minor.

Infections with the listed organisms are not always followed by abortion. Response may relate to route of access and involvement of fetus or membranes, the virulence of the organisms and size of inoculum, duration of maternal illness, degree of pyrexia and other reactions including prostaglandin synthesis.

Table 12.2. *Organisms associated with spontaneous abortion*

Viruses	
	Cytomegalovirus
	Herpes simplex
	Influenza
	Measles
	Mumps
	Parvo
	Polio
	Rubella
	Smallpox
Bacteria	
	Brucella abortus
	Campylobacter jejuni (Vibrio fetus)
	Haemophilus influenzae
	Leptospira icterohaemorrhagica
	Listeria monocytogenes
	Mycobacterium tuberculosis
	Salmonella spp.
	Treponema pallidum
Others	
	Candida spp.
	Chlamydia spp. (e.g. *Chlamydia psittaci* and *Chlamydia trachomatis*)
	Mycoplasma spp.
	Plasmodium spp.
	Toxoplasma gondii

Infection and fetal abnormality

The mechanisms whereby infections cause fetal damage may involve:

1. organisms proliferating preferentially in certain tissues, with cytolysis, inflammation and fibrosis;
2. alteration or arrest of organ development at critical phases, by vascular insufficiency due to damage to placental or fetal vessels;
3. maternal response to the presence of circulating organisms: maternal hyperthermia due to infection but also due to prolonged sauna bathing can be teratogenic, producing central nervous system dysfunction and facial dysmorphogenesis (25).

Although the role of infection cannot be ignored, it appears to account for only 1–2% of the total number of major congenital abnormalities (26, 27). Further, not every fetus exposed to a specific infection will become infected or show abnormal development. Prenatal diagnosis of cytomegalovirus, rubella and *Toxoplasma* infections is now available by fetal blood sampling and detection of specific IgM (28), and selective termination or appropriate antimicrobial therapy for toxoplasmosis may now be offered (29).

Infection and retardation of intrauterine growth, or fetal death

The factors which retard fetal growth are increasing in number and understanding, but infection must not be forgotten. The effect of certain viruses in producing small-for-dates infants is well recorded. The impact of other more frequently found organisms on fetal growth is not known.

Mechanisms are likely to be similar to those causing teratogenicity earlier in the pregnancy, but also include:

1. placentitis, when intervillous spaces are damaged or contain macrophages and organisms (as with malaria);
2. reduction in total number of cells in affected organs after some infections, such as rubella (17);
3. damage to one or several fetal organs by invading organisms, but with the insult modified by fetal immune response (cellular and immunoglobulin components appearing during the second trimester);
4. damage due to lifestyle and exposure to factors such as alcohol, cigarettes,

narcotics or inadequate diet, any or all of which may contribute to the growth retardation associated with infection by *Mycoplasma*, *Chlamydia* and other sexually transmitted agents.

The investigations that follow fetal death should include microbiological, histological and cytogenetic assessment of the fetus and placenta, fetal blood for IgM, and TORCH (*Toxoplasma*, rubella virus, cytomegalovirus and herpes simplex viruses) screening for maternal antibodies. Other organisms (listed in Table 12.1) may or may not be sought by the perinatal pathologist. Maternal health details around the time of fetal demise should include an extensive family and occupational history, animal contacts or food consumed, as well as details relevant to non-infective causes. Other infections recently seen within the hospital or area may have epidemiological significance. A retrospective diagnosis may be important in planning management for a subsequent pregnancy.

Infection and preterm labour

The factors which initiate the cascade of events responsible for the onset of labour still elude our understanding. However, there is no doubt that prostaglandins of the E and F groups play a key role. Arachidonic acid, the precursor of these prostaglandins, is produced at the interface between maternal decidua and fetal membrane, and is cleaved by certain enzymes including phospholipases. It is known that certain vaginal organisms including gram-negative bacilli and anaerobes can produce phospholipases (30). Alternatively, infection may produce chorioamnionitis or cervicitis, and thence release chemical mediators to stimulate prostaglandin production or release.

The presence of chorioamnionitis is difficult to interpret when the membranes have ruptured; ascending infection may quickly follow breach of the membranes. However, studies of the membranes and placenta can show histological evidence of chorioamnionitis after preterm labour with intact membranes (31).

Further evidence for the role of infection is seen in the infectious morbidity of the mother during the puerperium following preterm labour (32), and in the report that amniotic fluid contained higher levels of prostaglandins E and F when intra-amniotic infection was present (33).

Some of the organisms linked with preterm labour are listed in Table 12.1. Those organisms associated with phospholipase production include *Escherichia coli*, *Bacteroides* spp., enterococci, anaerobic streptococci, peptococci and *G. vaginalis*. It is uncertain whether high concentrations of a single organism within the vagina, as in bacterial vaginosis (34), or the combination of organisms, is important. The link between vaginal pH and preterm labour (35, 36) may be due to a reduction of some organisms, such as lactobacilli, allowing overgrowth of others.

The link between acute pyelonephritis and preterm labour (2) may be due to systemically released inflammation-associated mediators, as seen with acute peritonitis. Thomsen et al. (37) have suggested an alternative explanation: preterm labour linked with group B streptococcal bacteriuria may reflect the heaviness of bacterial colonization within the lower genital and urinary tracts.

Infection, and intrapartum transmission to the newborn

The flora of the vagina in late pregnancy consists of many organisms of low virulence, such as lactobacilli, *Staphylococcus epidermidis* and yeasts, and also small numbers of highly virulent organisms including *Staphy. aureus*, group A and B streptococci, enterococci, gram-negative bacilli, *Bacteroides* spp., *Clostridium* spp. and *Mycoplasma*. There may also be one or more sexually transmitted organisms including *Chlamydia*, *Neisseria* spp., and the human papilloma, hepatitis B, herpes simplex and human immunodeficiency viruses.

Factors which increase the risk of transmission to the neonate include the duration of the labour, duration of membrane rupture, and perhaps the number of vaginal examinations and the duration of fetal monitoring. Contamination from vulval or perineal organisms may occur in the second stage of labour, and in selected cases can be avoided by delivery by caesarean section (see section on screening for herpes simplex on p. 156).

Screening for infection during pregnancy

The value of screening will be influenced by the characteristics of the particular obstetric population and the prevalence of individual infections. It will depend on:

1. severity of infection, or its sequelae;
2. ability to recognize infection if it is present, or if it occurs during the pregnancy after the patient is found to be susceptible;
3. ability to treat infection if it is detected and thereby prevent sequelae or reduce perinatal morbidity.

Screening for a particular infection may be

1. appropriate for every antenatal patient;
2. appropriate for selected patients;
3. inappropriate (at present).

Screening generally takes place at booking, although there are exceptions (e.g. screening for genital tract infections, see later).

Screening in all antenatal patients

Rubella

The introduction of rubella vaccination has not produced total immunity in the population – some 3% of women of reproductive age remain susceptible (38). Screening is now by a single radial haemolysis technique against a standard of 15 iu. The current cost is 80 p per patient. Those susceptible should be vaccinated in the puerperium. If a patient reports contact, she can be reassured if immunity is present; if she is susceptible, further testing will be required. Screening for rubella status must continue, to assess efficacy of the new measles, mumps and rubella virus vaccination programme.

Syphilis

Screening for syphilis is still thought to be cost-effective, despite the current low prevalence of this infection in the heterosexual population in the UK. In 1987, 18 patients (0.5% of antenatal patients) at The Queen Mother's Hospital, Glasgow had a positive venereal disease research laboratory (VDRL) test and the *Treponema pallidum* haemagglutination test (TPHA) was positive in eight of these. All eight were known to have had previous infection, confirmed by IgG. More recently an enzyme-linked immunosorbant assay (ELISA) test has been introduced to give greater sensitivity and specificity than VDRL plus TPHA. This, however, will not detect the occasional patient with a false-positive VDRL due to the presence of lupus anticoagulant. Screening for syphilis should be performed early, to allow recognition and treatment before 16–20 weeks, thereby avoiding late sequelae.

Bacteriuria

Booking examination should include culture of a midstream specimen of urine. The use of a dipslide (39) provides simple, inexpensive

(31 p per specimen) quantitation of organisms present, with bacterial colonies suitable for subsequent antibiotic sensitivity testing.

Screening in selected patients

Varicella zoster virus

The majority of women who reach reproductive age have already been exposed to VZV and therefore have immunity. Most of those who are exposed to VZV during pregnancy either at home or in the community, will have definite recollection of childhood infection. Those who are uncertain should be tested for the presence of varicella antibody and, if seronegative, promptly receive varicella zoster immunoglobulin (40).

Human immunodeficiency virus

It can be argued that all antenatal patients should be screened for HIV infection, but currently compulsory testing is regarded as unethical (41). A second approach is to ask antenatal patients to volunteer to be tested; such a programme is being assessed in Edinburgh, Dundee and elsewhere. A recently reported study from London (42) found that 26% of patients declined the offered test. It is likely that those who decline include some who fear that they have already been exposed to the infection. Whole-population screening can be applied to the newborn population by testing the HIV antibody status of dried blood obtained for Guthrie testing for inherited metabolic disease. A further approach is to identify women at high risk of encountering the infection, and offer them testing.

Table 12.3 shows the information sheet that is sent now to all patients prior to their booking visit at The Queen Mother's Hospital, Glasgow. This list is similar to that advised by the Royal College of Obstetricians and Gynaecologists. Patients are asked to identify themselves if they believe they are at risk of infection. The only specific question that is asked at booking is whether the woman or her partner have used drugs. In the light of recent revelations it may also be relevant to ask if the women or her partner has been in prison recently.

If the antenatal patient identifies herself as at risk, she should be given pretest information:

1. the test is a blood test;
2. the chances of a false-positive test are very small;

Table 12.3. *Information sheet on risk factors for infection with human immunodeficiency virus (HIV) (The Queen Mother's Hospital, Glasgow)*

Currently, The Queen Mother's Hospital does not screen every patient for HIV infection (AIDS). However, it is recognized that this infection may produce an adverse outcome for mothers and their babies. The following are thought to increase your risk of infection:

1. if you or your partner has had a blood transfusion, outside the United Kingdom, since 1980
2. if your partner is haemophiliac
3. if you or your partner has had sex at any time with someone living in Central African countries, Haiti, certain areas of the United States of America, including California, or from cities within Italy, Spain, Portugal and Holland
4. if you or your partner has injected drugs
5. if your partner is bisexual
6. if you or your partner has been involved in casual sexual associations or prostitution

If you believe that one of these factors may place you at risk, you are advised to tell your obstetrician at the time of your booking visit. This information will be treated confidentially. After counselling, you will be offered a blood test for HIV infection. No one will be tested without consent.

3. a negative test does not necessarily exclude HIV infection and repeat testing may be required;
4. if the test is positive, further counselling regarding the risk to the woman during her pregnancy and to her infant will be required; in some circumstances, termination of pregnancy may be recommended;
5. the result will be notified by interview, and not by letter or telephone;
6. the woman has the choice of notifying her general practitioner of the result;
7. the woman has the choice of notifying her partner of the result;
8. medical support and counsellors are available if the result is positive;
9. a positive result will require careful planning of further health care, including management of the pregnancy and infant;
10. if the result is negative, the woman should take appropriate measures to reduce risk activities.

Following receipt of this information the woman should sign an appropriate form, consenting to be tested. A patient with a positive test requires counselling by a health team who understand the management problems in pregnancy as well as subsequently.

Hepatitis B

The incidence of hepatitis B viral infection is increasing in the UK. Between 2 and 4% of the population have serological evidence of exposure, and 0.1% are carriers (43). However, people coming from endemic areas will have a much greater risk of being infected. Therefore current practice is to screen only selected antenatal patients. Those at risk include those at risk of HIV infection (Table 12.3) plus:

1. those from endemic areas, and this list includes most of the world except Europe, North America and Australia (or their partners);
2. those exposed to blood products, such as dialysis patients (or their partners);
3. inmates from prisons (or their partners);
4. those with acute or chronic liver disease.

The recognition of hepatitis B in an antenatal patient enables appropriate steps to be taken to protect staff, and to protect the neonate.

Tuberculosis

Screening for tuberculosis in pregnancy is no longer done as a routine, but is carried out in selected patients:

1. immigrants from developing countries or those recently visiting/resident in high-risk countries;
2. those with recent family tuberculosis contact;
3. those with respiratory symptoms or recurrent fever that fails to respond to standard antibiotic therapy.

Screening should be by chest X-ray and Mantoux testing.

Toxoplasmosis

Screening for toxoplasmosis is not performed within the UK, but is done elsewhere in Europe where the risks for infection are believed to be greater (France, Belgium, Austria, Germany and Italy). In a study carried out in Glasgow on samples collected between 1975 and 1977 a seroconversion rate of 2.3 per 1000 pregnancies was reported in women previously without antibody (44). Seroconversion during pregnancy is 10 per 1000 in France, 8.5 per 1000 in Austria and 6 per 1000 in Germany. Maternal toxoplasmosis is usually asymptomatic. Screening would involve testing (Sabin–Feldman dye test, fluorescent antibody test, complement fixation or haemagglutination tests) all women at booking, and retesting all seronegative patients (approximately 75% of the total) at intervals for evidence of seroconversion. Transmission of infection to the fetus will occur in approximately 45% of mothers who seroconvert (45). The classic triad of manifestations is chorioretinitis, hydrocephalus and intracranial calcification. Diagnosis of fetal infection is by isolation of the parasite following inoculation of liquor (from amniocentesis) or fetal blood (from cordocentesis) into mice. A fetal blood sample can also be examined for *Toxoplasma*-specific IgM (28) and for eosinophilia, thrombocytopaenia and abnormal hepatic enzymes. Ultrasound scanning for ventricular dilatation may be useful. However, only 10–20% of congenitally infected infants will have clinically apparent disease at birth: the others are still at risk of developing manifestations some time later (46). Termination of pregnancy does not seem justified if seroconversion occurs, but prenatal therapy with spiramycin or sulphonamide–pyrimethamine appears valuable while awaiting fetal blood and inoculation results (29).

Genital tract infection

Recent studies have reported that *Chlamydia trachomatis* may be found in up to 7% of antenatal patients (47). The likelihood of infection cannot be predicted from genital symptoms. As the consequences of this infection are significant for the neonate and as effective screening tests are now available, consideration must be given to screening for this infection. This is better done in the third trimester rather than at booking.

In a study reported from New Zealand in 1977 (1) the incidence of gonorrhoea found at booking clinic examination was 1.3% for unmarried women and 0.4% for married women. However, it is no longer appropriate to use marital status to designate risk. As with *Chlamydia* infection, the majority of pregnant women infected by neisseria will be asymptomatic. As *Neisseria gonorrhoeae* can be isolated from various sites, infection may be missed if only the cervix is swabbed. Current prevalence of gonorrhoea in the UK does not justify routine antenatal screening.

It is not unusual for trichomonads to be identified in cervical smears taken at booking visit. However, there is no evidence to link trichomoniasis with abortion, preterm labour or transmission to the neonate. The infection need only be treated if the patient is symptomatic, and then with vaginal cream or pessary rather than oral therapy.

Candida is frequently identified during pregnancy, and can cause fetal infection or be transmitted to the neonate. However, current practice is not to screen, and to treat only those patients who have vulvitis.

Human papillomavirus is widely found in the genital tract, and can be transmitted to the neonate. Estimates of the risk of laryngeal papillomata developing in children born to women with vulval condylomata vary between 1 in 80 and 1 in 1500, based on a survey by North American otolaryngologists (48). Although there are those who would justify treatment of condylomata during pregnancy to avoid this risk (49), most British obstetricians would only provide treatment if there was concern that the lesion might complicate vaginal delivery. As HPV DNA can be identified, using polymerase chain reaction techniques, in up to 84% of normal cervices (50) and as currently there is no effective treatment to eradicate this virus from the genital tract, screening for HPV is not justified.

Screening for herpes simplex virus has concentrated on those with a previous history of infection. Previously, viral swabs were taken at weekly intervals from 36 weeks for evidence of viral shedding. When the patient was admitted in labour, with a known positive swab from the previous week, and the membranes were intact or ruptured for no more than 4 h, she was sectioned; otherwise vaginal delivery was allowed. However, this policy has been questioned (27, 51), as maternal antibodies from a previous infection appear to protect the neonate, and many patients have had unnecessary sections. The greatest neonatal risk occurs with primary maternal infection, with a transmission risk of 50%. Therefore screening now seems unjustified, but any woman with clinical lesions at the onset of labour should be delivered by caesarean section (52).

As a significant number of pregnant women can carry *Listeria* in their intestine, but rarely in the vagina, there appears to be no value in screening for *Listeria*.

Attempts have been made to correlate preterm labour with the presence of specific organisms (see earlier). There may be a correlation between some of these organisms, vaginal pH and preterm labour (35, 36), but currently it does not justify screening.

Infections for which screening is currently inappropriate

Cytomegalovirus

The sequelae of cytomegalovirus infection for the fetus are described elsewhere. The consensus (27, 53) is that screening for infection during pregnancy is not justified, because:

1. the presence of maternal antibodies is not protective and reinfection can produce fetal damage;
2. maternal infection is usually asymptomatic and most diagnoses are made only retrospectively;
3. termination of pregnancy is not justified after seroconversion, and fetal damage from exposure to infection can occur in any trimester;
4. unlike rubella, there is no effective vaccine to offer postnatally to those patients who are seronegative;
5. no suitable antiviral agent is available for administration during pregnancy.

Group A and B streptococci

Beta-haemolytic streptococci are subdivided into Lancefield groups. Group A includes *Streptococcus pyogenes*, the organism of childbed fever, and this is found in less than 1% of genital tracts during pregnancy. Group B streptococci, or *Str. agalactiae*, are found in up to one-third of pregnant women. The incidence is greatest in young women of low parity, and those who are unbooked or book late. Approximately one in three of infants born to women with group B streptococci will themselves be colonized, but only 0.3 per 1000 liveborn infants in the UK develop early-onset disease. The problems in identifying the organisms include:

1. only 10% of organisms are recovered from swabs;
2. broth-enrichment techniques are necessary;
3. a single swab is inadequate – cervical swabs will detect only 30% of carriers, compared to an isolation rate from anorectal swabs of 80%;
4. carriage is intermittent or transitory, and swabbing on more than one occasion in the third trimester increases isolation rates (54).

Therefore screening for group B streptococcal carriage is not justified: to prevent one case of early-onset neonatal disease, 3000 women would need to be screened, and up to 1000 treated (55). An alternative, though equally unsatisfactory, approach is to treat every patient in labour.

A working compromise is to take swabs

from all women who present with preterm labour, preterm membrane rupture or multiple pregnancy in the third trimester. Those who have group B streptococci should be given intravenous penicillin during subsequent labour.

Antenatal infection has consequences for the mother and her fetus. The clinician must be alert to its presence, understand its manifestations, and know of its management.

References

1. MacLean AB, Paltridge S, Platts WM. Antenatal screening for gonorrhoea in Christchurch. NZ Med J 1977; 85: 136–8.
2. Kass EH. Maternal infections as affecting the outcome of pregnancy. NY State J Med 1962; 62: 2822–6.
3. Harris JW. Influenza occurring in pregnant women. J Am Med Assoc 1919; 72: 978–80.
4. Khuroo MS, Teli MR, Skidmore S, Sofi MA, Khuroo MI. Incidence and severity of viral hepatitis in pregnancy. Am J Med 1981; 70: 252–5.
5. Paryani SG, Arvin AM. Intrauterine infection with varicella-zoster virus after maternal varicella. N Engl J Med 1986; 314: 1542–6.
6. Kingdom JCP, Kennedy DH. Tuberculous meningitis in pregnancy. Br J Obstet Gynaecol 1989; 96: 233–5.
7. Vleugels MPH, Eling WMC, Rolland R, DeGraaf R. Cortisol and loss of malaria immunity in human pregnancy. Br J Obstet Gynaecol 1987; 94: 758–64.
8. Pinching AJ, Jeffries DJ. AIDS and HTLV-III/LAV infection: consequences for obstetrics and perinatal medicine. Br J Obstet Gynaecol 1985; 92: 1211–17.
9. Johnstone FD, Mok J. HIV infection. In: MacLean AB (ed) Clinical infection in obstetrics and gynaecology. Oxford: Blackwell Scientific 1990 pp 72–94.
10. Jones WR, Hawes CS, Kemp AS. Studies on cell-mediated immunity in human pregnancy. In: Wegman TG, Gill TJ (eds) Immunology of reproduction. Oxford: Oxford University Press, 1983: 365–80.
11. Ritz J. The role of natural killer cells in immune surveillance. Engl J Med 1989; 320: 1748–9.
12. Kurashige T, Morita H, Ogura H, Kurashige M, Kitamura I, Kamimura O. Natural killer cell activity in pregnancy and the effect of pregnant women's sera. Asia Oceania J Obstet Gynaecol 1986; 12: 305–9.
13. Sridama V, Pacini F, Yang S-L, Moawad A, Reilly M, DeGroot LJ. Decreased levels of helper T cells: a possible cause of immunodeficiency in pregnancy. N Engl J Med 1982; 397: 352–6.
14. Baboonian C, Griffiths P. Is pregnancy immunosuppressive? Humoral immunity against viruses. Br J Obstet Gynaecol 1983; 90: 1168–75.
15. Fox H. Infection of the placenta. In Fox H (ed) Pathology of the placenta. London: WB Saunders, 1978: 286–325.
16. Stray-Pedersen B, Eng J, Reikvam TM. Uterine T-mycoplasma colonisation in reproductive failure. Am J Obstet Gynecol 1978; 130: 307–11.
17. Naeye RL, Tafari N. Risk factors in pregnancy and diseases of the fetus and newborn. Baltimore: Williams and Wilkins, 1983: 19–75 and 77–143.
18. Alger LS, Lovchik JC, Hebel JR, Blackmon LR, Crenshaw MC. The association of *Chlamydia trachomatis*, *Neisseria gonorrhoeae*, and group B streptococci with preterm rupture of the membranes and pregnancy outcome. Am J Obstet Gynecol 1988; 159: 397–404.
19. Jackson LG, Wapner RJ. Risks of chorion villus sampling. Clin Obstet Gynaecol 1987; 1: 513–31.
20. Reed CS, Fledman RG, Cochrane RM. Amnionitis caused by *Propionibacterium acne*. Br J Obstet Gynaecol 1988; 95: 626–7.
21. Alvior GT. Pregnancy outcome with removal of intrauterine devices. Obstet Gynecol 1973; 41: 894–6.
22. Huisjes HJ. Spontaneous abortion. London: Churchill Livingstone, 1984.
23. Gronroos M, Honkonen E, Terho P, Punnonen R. Cervical and serum IgA and serum IgG antibodies to *Chlamydia trachomatis* and herpes simplex virus in threatened abortion: a prospective study. Br J Obstet Gynaecol 1983; 90: 167–70.
24. Munday PE, Porter R, Falder PF, Carder JM, Holliman R, Lewis BV, Taylor-Robinson D. Spontaneous abortion: an infectious aetiology? Br J Obstet Gynaecol 1984; 91: 1177–80.
25. Pleet H, Graham JM, Smith DW. Central nervous system and facial defects associated

with maternal hyperthermia at four to fourteen weeks' gestation. Pediatrics 1981; 67: 785–9.
26. Kalter H, Warkany J. Congenital malformations: etiologic factors and their role in prevention. N Engl J Med 1983; 308: 424–31.
27. Rudd P, Peckham C. Infection of the fetus and the newborn: prevention, treatment and related handicap. Clin Obstet Gynaecol 1988; 2: 55–71.
28. Nicolaides KH, Rodeck CH. Fetal blood sampling. Clin Obstet Gynaecol 1987; 1: 623–48.
29. Daffos F, Forestier F, Capella-Pavlovsky M, Thulliez P, Aufrant C, Valenti D, Cox WL. Prenatal management of 746 pregnancies at risk for congenital toxoplasmosis. N Engl J Med 1988; 318: 271–5.
30. Lamont RF, Rose M, Elder MG. Effect of bacterial products on prostaglandin E production by amnion cells. Lancet 1985; 2: 1331–3.
31. Harvey J, Agustsson P, Patel N, Anderson J. The role of infection in the aetiology of preterm labour. In: Beard RW, Sharp F (eds) Preterm labour and its consequences. Proceedings of the Thirteen Study Group of the Royal College of Obstetricians and Gynaecologists. London: RCOG, 1985: 249–58.
32. Daikoku NH, Kaltreider F, Khouzami VA, Spence M, Johnson JWC. Premature rupture of membranes and spontaneous preterm labour: maternal endometritis risks. Obstet Gynecol 1982; 59: 13–20.
33. Romero R, Emamian M, Quintero R, Wan M, Hobbins JC, Mitchell MD. Amniotic fluid prostaglandin levels and intra-amniotic infections. Lancet 1986; 1: 1380.
34. Eschenbach DA, Gravett MG, Chen KCS, Hoyme UB, Holmes KK. Bacterial vaginosis during pregnancy. Scand J Urol Nephrol 1984; 86: 213–22.
35. Minkoff H, Grunebaum A, Feldman J, Cumming M, McCormack WM. Relationship of vaginal pH and Papanicolaou smear results to vaginal flora and pregnancy outcome. Int J Gynaecol Obstet 1987; 25: 17–23.
36. Gleeson RP, Elder AM, Turner MJ, Rutherford AJ, Elder MG. Vaginal pH in pregnancy in women delivered at and before term. Br J Obstet Gynaecol 1989; 96: 183–7.
37. Thomsen AC, Morup L, Hansen KB. Antibiotic elimination of group B streptococci in urine in prevention of preterm labour. Lancet 1987; 2: 591–3.
38. Noah ND, Fowle SE. Immunity to rubella in women in childbearing age in the United Kingdom. Br Med J 1988; 297: 1301–4.
39. McAllister TA. The day of the dipslide. Nephron 1973; 11: 123–33.
40. McGregor JA, Mark S, Crawford GP, Levin MJ. Varicella zoster antibody testing in the care of pregnant women exposed to varicella. Am J Obstet Gynecol 1987; 157: 281–4.
41. Howie PW. Antenatal HIV screening: ethical considerations. In: Hudson CN, Sharp F (eds) AIDS and obstetrics and gynaecology. London: Royal College of Obstetricians and Gynaecologists, 1988: 127–32.
42. Howard LC, Hawkins DA, Marwood R, Shanson DC, Gazzard BG. Transmission of human immunodeficiency virus by heterosexual contact with reference to antenatal screening. Br J Obstet Gynaecol 1989; 96: 135–9.
43. Finch RG. Time for action on hepatitis B immunisation. Br Med J 1987; 294: 197–9.
44. Williams KAB, Scott JM, Macfarlane DE, Williamson JMW, Elias-Jones TF, Williams H. Congenital toxoplasmosis; a prospective survey in the West of Scotland. J Infect 1981; 3: 219–29.
45. Stray-Pedersen B. A prospective study of acquired toxoplasmosis among 8043 pregnant women in the Oslo area. Am J Obstet Gynecol 1980; 136: 399–406.
46. Hall SM. Congenital toxoplasmosis in England, Wales and Northern Ireland: some epidemiological problems. Br Med J 1983; 287: 453–5.
47. Wood PL, Hobson D, Rees E. Genital infections with *Chlamydia trachomatis* in women attending an antenatal clinic. Br J Obstet Gynaecol 1984; 91: 1171–6.
48. Shah K, Kashima H, Polk BF, Shah F, Abbey H, Abramson A. Rarity of cesarean delivery in cases of juvenile-onset respiratory papillomatosis. Obstet Gynecol 1986; 68: 795–9.
49. Schwartz DB, Greenberg MD, Daoud Y, Reid R. Genital condylomas in pregnancy: use of trichloroacetic acid and laser therapy. Am J Obstet Gynecol 1988; 158: 1407–16.
50. Tidy JA, Parry GCN, Ward P, Coleman DV, Peto J, Malcolm ADB, Farrell PJ. High rate of human papillomavirus type 16 infection in cytologically normal cervices. Lancet 1989; i: 434.
51. Prober CG, Sullender WM, Yasukawa LL, Au DS, Yeoger A, Arvin AM. Low risk of herpes simplex virus infections in neonates exposed

to the virus at the time of vaginal delivery to mothers with recurrent genital herpes simplex virus infection. N Engl J Med 1987; 316: 240–4.
52. Editorial. Virological screening for herpes simplex virus during pregnancy. Lancet 1988; 2: 722–3.
53. Jeffries DJ. Cytomegalovirus infections in pregnancy. Br J Obstet Gynaecol 1984; 91: 305–6.
54. Ross PW. Group B streptococcus: profile of an organism. J Med Microbiol 1984; 18: 139–44.
55. Easmon CSF, Hastings MJG, Neill J, Bloxham B, Rivers PRA. Is group B streptococcal screening during pregnancy justified? Br J Obstet Gynaecol 1985; 92: 197–201.

Index